The Best Foods for Diabetes

100 Easy, Delicious And Mouthwatering Superfoods to Reverse Diabetes And Lower Blood Sugar - The Smart Blood Sugar Solution

Kimberly Mays

Digital Print House Inc

© Copyright 2017 by - Digital Print House Inc - All rights reserved.

This document is geared toward providing exact and reliable information in regards to the topic and issue covered. The publication is sold with the idea that the publisher is not required to render accounting, officially permitted, or otherwise qualified services. If advice is necessary, legal or professional, a practiced individual in the profession should be ordered.

From a Declaration of Principles which was accepted and approved equally by a Committee of the American Bar Association and a Committee of Publishers and Associations.

In no way is it legal to reproduce, duplicate, or transmit any part of this document in either electronic means or in printed format. Recording of this publication is strictly prohibited and any storage of this document is not allowed unless with written permission from the publisher. All rights reserved.

The information provided herein is stated to be truthful and consistent, in that any liability, in terms of inattention or otherwise, by any usage or abuse of any policies, processes, or directions contained within is the solitary and utter responsibility of the recipient reader. Under no circumstances will any legal responsibility or blame be held against the publisher for any reparation, damages, or monetary loss due to the information herein, either directly or indirectly.

Respective authors own all copyrights not held by the publisher.

The information herein is offered for informational purposes solely, and is universal as so. The presentation of the information is without contract or any type of guarantee assurance.

The trademarks that are used are without any consent, and the publication of the trademark is without permission or backing by the trademark owner. All trademarks and brands within this book are for clarifying purposes only and are owned by the owners themselves, not affiliated with this document.

Table of Contents

Introduction 1

Chapter 1: The Basics of a Diabetes Diet 3

Chapter 2: Diabetes Super Foods 7

Chapter 3: All About Dessert 11

Chapter 4: Stocking the Pantry 15

Chapter 5: 100 Diabetes-Friendly Recipes 19

    Breakfast 19

    Drinks & Smoothies 45

    Berry-Oat Smoothie 47

    Soups & Stews 55

    Main Dishes 76

    Slow Cooker Recipes 107

    Vegetables & Sides 131

    Desserts 163

    Snacks 191

    Pantry Staples 208

Takeaways 221

One Last Thought 223

Resources Cited 225

YOUR FREE BONUS

Download Another Book for Free

I want to thank you for buying this book and assist you even further in your quest to a better health by giving you **free, instant access to this cookbook with over 500 delicious Diabetic Recipes.**

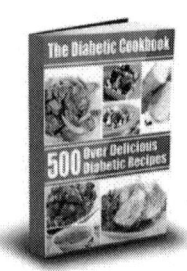

"Get FREE Instant Access To Over 500 Delicious Diabetic Recipes In This Amazing Diabetic Cookbook + FREE Tips for a Diabetes Diet Email Series [$97 Value]

When you sign up today, you Get all the above plus FREE Subscriber-only Diabetes diet advice, tips and tricks via email including a FREE Weight loss and exercise for Diabetes report. Get instant access now

Download Now!

Get My Free Report Now!

Download your free cookbook at:

https://rock85.leadpages.co/diabetes-recepies-/

Introduction

Diabetes is one of the leading health problems in the country. According to some studies, more than 29 million Americans have diabetes. Of those, one in four may not even be aware of their condition. In addition to the number of Americans with diabetes, many more are at risk. One out of every three adults has prediabetes.[1] Whether you have diabetes or prediabetes or are simply concerned for a family member or friend, this book will teach you the basics of selecting foods and recipes for a diabetes diet.

You can still enjoy your favorite foods with diabetes.

YES, even dessert!

Cooking with diabetes does not need to be a stressful experience. By making a plan and learning to adapt your favorite recipes to be diabetes-friendly, you can make the transition painlessly. This book will teach you how to cook meals that the entire family can enjoy without exceeding the nutritional recommendations of your doctor or dietician. Now is the time to learn about cooking with diabetes, whether for yourself or a loved one.

In this book, you will learn more about the foods to eat and those to avoid. You will find tricks for making the most of the sugar you do eat and multiple ways to plan your diet, including on

---

[1] "Diabetes Latest." National Center for Chronic Disease Prevention and Health Promotion, 2014: https://www.cdc.gov/features/diabetesfactsheet/

special occasions and days when dessert is a part of the plan. No matter your background in the kitchen, you will find recipes to suit your tastes and schedule. With 100 diabetes-friendly recipes, including desserts, breakfast foods, and slow cooker recipes, you are sure to discover a new family favorite.

Chapter 1

The Basics of a Diabetes Diet

Understanding how food affects your blood sugar should be the first part of any diabetes diet plan.

One of the most important parts of a diabetes diet is having a plan. There are multiple ways to track your diet. Two of the most common are the glycemic index and diabetes food exchanges. Here are a few basics you need to know about each:

Glycemic Index

The glycemic index is a number given to foods that identifies how much it will affect your blood sugar level. Higher numbers are given to foods that raise blood glucose levels more than those with lower numbers. It is not necessary to completely eliminate foods high on the glycemic index, although they will require more planning than those low on the index. With some planning, the glycemic index can provide a great guideline on what foods to combine for best results. Examples of foods high on the glycemic index are white bread, white rice, popcorn, white potatoes, and watermelon. Foods low on the glycemic index include whole wheat bread, peas, lentils, oatmeal, and barley.

Exchanges

A diabetes exchange diet works on universal principles of solid nutrition. Exchange lists divide foods into six groups: starch/bread, meat, vegetable, fruit, milk, and fat. Foods are arranged in each list by their basic nutritional components. This organization makes it

Chapter 2

Diabetes Super Foods

Some foods have a positive effect on blood sugar levels. Increasing your intake of these foods can help control your diabetes.

Cinnamon

After analyzing three different medical studies involving cinnamon consumption in patients with type 2 diabetes or prediabetes, Davis and Yokoyama (2011) indicated that both whole cinnamon and cinnamon extract reduce the fasting blood glucose levels of patients with type 2 diabetes and prediabetes.[2] Cinnamon is especially beneficial because it is relatively inexpensive and easy to find. It is also extremely versatile; cinnamon pairs well with baked goods, desserts, and savory dishes. Sprinkle cinnamon on your morning.

Fenugreek Seeds

Fenugreek seeds have been used medicinally for centuries. Recent research supports the claim that fenugreek seeds can reduce fasting blood sugar levels. A study by Sharma et al. (1990) found that regular consumption of fenugreek seed powder lowered cholesterol and triglyceride levels as well.[3] The fiber in fenugreek seeds slows the body's absorption of sugar. Fenugreek

---

[2] Davis PA & Yokoyama W (2011) Cinnamon intake lowers fasting blood glucose: meta analysis. J Med Food 14:884-889.
[3] Sharma RD, Raghuram TC, & Rao NS (1990) Effect of fenugreek seeds on blood glucose and serum lipids in type 1 diabetes. Eur J Clin Nutr 44:301-306.

seeds can be used as seasoning in curry, pickle brine, tea, or baked goods. When it comes to working fenugreek seeds into your diabetes diet, research done by Kassaian et al. (2009) found a more significant result in study participants who consumed fenugreek seeds after steeping in hot water than those who ate them raw in yogurt—yet another benefit to fenugreek tea.[4]

Avocado

Healthy fats are a great way to keep your blood sugar from spiking and keep your energy up all day. Avocados are high in monounsaturated fat—one of the healthiest fats. They are also low in sugar. Both of these characteristics are beneficial for heart health. Because people with diabetes are at risk for heart disease, this is an especially important benefit. Avocados' creamy texture makes them an easy substitute for mayonnaise or other spreads.

Leafy Greens

Nearly all dieticians and doctors agree that we should be eating more leafy green vegetables. Leafy greens like kale, chard, and spinach are high in fiber, which helps control blood sugar. Leafy green vegetables are also high in vitamins A, B, C, and K in addition to having high amounts of iron and protein. Finding a way to eat more leafy green vegetables will go a long way to controlling your blood sugar. Many greens can be eaten raw in a

---

[4] Kassaian N, Azadbakht L, Forghani B, & Amini M (2009) Effect of fenugreek seeds on blood glucose and lipid profiles in type 2 diabetes patients. Int J Vitam Nutr Res 79: 34-39.

salad, while some of the more fibrous greens are best braised or steamed.

Yogurt

One of the main reasons yogurt is beneficial for a diabetes diet is because the high protein content of yogurt helps control cravings throughout the day. In addition to its protein content, the probiotics in yogurt can improve appetite control and reduce inflammation. According to Ejtahed et al. (2012), probiotic yogurt improves fasting glucose levels in patients with type 2 diabetes.[5] Substitute yogurt for sour cream in your favorite recipes or eat it with fresh granola for a mid-day snack. When incorporating yogurt into your diet, however, be sure to check the nutrition labels. Many commercial yogurts contain added sweeteners and not all brands are sweetened equally. Plain yogurt can be sweetened at home to taste with honey or maple syrup. Greek yogurt is even higher in protein than traditional yogurt, making it a satisfying and filling option.

Lentils

Lentils are a great source of fiber and protein. They are low on the glycemic index and can be included in many types of foods. Beans and lentils are inexpensive ways to eat your fill. In addition to being high in fiber and low on the glycemic index, lentils are full of B vitamins, iron, and protein. Lentils are related to beans

---

[5] Ejtahed HS, Mohtadi-Nia J, Homayouni-Rad A, Niafar M, Asghari-Jafarabadi M, & Mofid V (2012) Probiotic yogurt improves antioxidant status in type 2 diabetes patients. Nutrition 28:539-543.

(they are both legumes) but have some distinct advantages of their own. Lentils do not need to be soaked overnight before using, unlike many dried beans. They can be added to ground beef mixtures to make the meat go further, which can be great for the budget and for your blood glucose levels. Brown and green lentils have a nutty taste and firmer texture, while red lentils are softer and make great additions to soups and purees.

Chapter 2 Takeaways

1. Some foods are easier to incorporate into a diabetes diet than others. The super foods on this list have extra benefits for people watching their blood sugar levels.

2. Look for foods that are high in fiber and protein, like lentils and leafy greens.

3. Not all fats are created equally—full-fat yogurt and avocados are both good for your heart and blood glucose levels.

Chapter 3

All About Dessert

There are a number of easy ways you can enjoy your favorite desserts and still meet your diet goals.

Dessert needs not be forbidden on a diabetes diet! Portion control and moderation are two easy ways to include your favorite desserts in your diet plan. When figuring out your daily or weekly diet, account for dessert as you plan your meals. Remember that most desserts will not contain vitamins and nutrients that your body needs, so be sure to eat foods higher in those essential nutrients on days when you plan to eat dessert. Here are three suggestions for successfully working dessert into your plan:

1. *Stick to smaller portions of your favorite desserts.* A little can also go a long way—miniature chocolate chips, for example, give you a little chocolate in every bite without the sugar count of regular chocolate chips.

2. *Make dessert a special occasion.* Eating something sweet after dinner may have become more of a habit than you realize, but not every meal must end with a sweet bite. In many cases, you may just need to eat more dinner. Something cold can substitute for something sweet if you need a contrast to a savory meal. By breaking the habit of nightly dessert, you will find your favorite treats fit in your nutritional goals more easily.

3. *Consider a sugar substitute.* Reducing the amount of sugar you eat is the best way to control your blood sugar, but sugar substitutes are another option for cooking with diabetes. Splenda and

other sucralose products are much sweeter than regular sugar, so start small. The chemical aftertaste makes Splenda difficult for baking, but it works very well in coffee and other strong drinks. Saccharin (often sold under the name Sweet'n Low) is another calorie-free sweetener that is much stronger than regular sugar. Some research has indicated that saccharin can lead to weight gain, however, so it should be used sparingly. Stevia sweeteners are extracted from the leaf of the stevia plant and have very little impact on blood sugars. Commercial stevia blends are available specifically for baking as well, making it easier to use in much-loved family recipes.

The Difference in Low-Sugar Cooking

When you reduce the amount of sugar in your favorite recipes or begin trying new diabetes-friendly recipes, you may notice some differences in your finished product:

1. *Your baked goods will not brown as easily.* Browning is a result of the caramelization of sugars. Cookies and breads may be completely baked but not the color you expect. An egg wash or higher baking temperature can counteract this effect.

2. *Breads get stale faster.* Without extra sugars, your homemade breads may get stale faster than commercial breads. You can combat this by slicing and freezing extra loaves and thawing slices one at a time when you are ready for them.

3. *Ice creams and sorbets will be less creamy.* The best thing about making homemade ice creams and sorbets is that you will still be able to enjoy many of your favorite frozen treats. Less

sugar will result in a slightly less creamy product, however, which can be mitigated by thoroughly chilling all ingredients before churning the ice cream. Smaller ice crystals will lead to a smoother ice cream.

4. *Make the most of the sugar you do use.* Many recipes contain more sugar than they need. Start by reducing the sugar by a third. Try sprinkling sugar on top of muffins and cookies. It can give more sweetness for the amount of sugar used. The same is true of powdered or confectioner's sugar—a small dusting of powdered sugar can make foods seem like a treat without adding too many extra sugars.

Chapter 3 Takeaways

1. Treat yourself to a smaller portion of your favorite desserts rather than filling up on less-satisfying replacements.

2. Look for a special baking blend when using sugar substitutes in your favorite recipes.

3. Using a small amount of sugar on top of baked goods can make them seem much sweeter without using the full sugar called for in the recipe. Keep a shaker of cinnamon sugar or powdered sugar on hand for topping muffins and more.

Chapter 4

Stocking the Pantry

A well-stocked pantry will help you stick to your plan.

In addition to the super foods discussed previously, here is a list of foods to keep on hand for easy snacking and baking:

Grains

- whole grain pasta
- brown rice
- oatmeal (rolled oats and steel cut)
- quinoa

Beans and Legumes

- canned beans
- dried beans
- lentils
- dried peas

Fats and Oils

- coconut oil
- extra virgin olive oil
- balsamic vinegar

- flavored oils and vinegar

Dry Goods

- sugar substitute (baking blend)
- low-sugar spice blends
- low-sugar ketchup
- sugar-free mayonnaise
- low-sugar salad dressing
- canned fish
- all-natural nut butter
- mini chocolate chips
- raw pecans, almonds, and walnuts
- high-quality chicken stock

Cold Items

- frozen edamame
- pastured eggs
- unsweetened almond milk
- plain yogurt
- cream cheese
- hummus

Chapter 4 Takeaways

1. Keep a combination of quick snacks and meal ingredients in the house to prevent impulse snacking and fast food visits.

2. Focus on ingredients that are high in flavor without the sugar or fat: dried and fresh herbs, flavored oils, vinegar, etc.

3. When possible, purchase or make low-or no-sugar condiments and sauces.

Chapter 5

100 Diabetes-Friendly Recipes

With everything from breakfast to dessert, these 100 diabetes-friendly recipes are sure to be a hit for you and yours.

Breakfast
Whole Wheat Oat Bran Muffins

Prep Time: 10 minutes

Cook Time: 20 minutes

Yield: 12 muffins

Ingredients:

- 3/4 c. whole wheat flour
- 1 1/4 c. oat bran
- 1 tsp. baking soda
- 1/2 tsp. ground cinnamon
- 1/2 tsp. kosher salt
- 1/3 c. brown sugar
- 1/4 c. coconut oil, melted
- 1 c. buttermilk
- 1 egg, beaten
- 1 tsp. vanilla extract

Directions:

Preheat the oven to 375°F. In a large boil, combine flour, bran, soda, cinnamon, and salt. Set aside. Whisk sugar, coconut oil, buttermilk, egg, and vanilla together in another bowl. Pour wet ingredients into dry ingredients and fold until just combined, being careful not to over mix. Spoon batter evenly into greased or lined muffin cups, filling each cup 2/3 full. Bake for 15-28 minutes.

Nutritional Information:

- Calories: 104.1
- Fat: 5.5g
- Cholesterol: 16.3mg
- Sodium: 214mg
- Potassium: 72.4mg
- Carbohydrates: 14.6g
- Dietary Fiber: 1.6g
- Sugars: 6.4g
- Protein: 2.9g

Nutty Granola

Prep Time: 10 minutes

Cook Time: 75 minutes

Yield: 10 servings

Ingredients:

- 3 c. rolled oats
- 1 c. sliced or slivered almonds
- 1/2 c. walnuts, roughly chopped
- 1/2 c. pecans, roughly chopped
- 1/4 c. raw sunflower seeds
- 3 T. ground flax seed meal
- 3 T. chia seeds
- 3 T. sesame seeds
- 1/2 c. coconut oil, melted
- 2 T. raw honey
- 1/2 tsp. kosher salt

Directions:

Preheat oven to 250°F. Line two sheet pans with parchment paper and set aside. In a large bowl, combine oats, almonds, walnuts, pecans, sunflower seeds, flax seed meal, chia seeds, and sesame seeds. In another bowl, combine coconut oil, honey, and salt. Stir together both mixtures and spread evenly between sheet pans. Bake for 75 minutes, stirring twice and rotating the position of the pans in the oven once. Allow the granola to cool on the pan completely before breaking into chunks. Any combination of nuts and seeds can be used to accommodate allergies or personal preference as long as the overall volume remains the same.

Nutritional Information:

- Calories: 382.6
- Fat: 29.5g
- Cholesterol: 0mg
- Sodium: 96.4mg
- Potassium: 183mg
- Carbohydrates: 26.5g
- Dietary Fiber: 7.2g
- Sugars: 4.9g
- Protein: 8.7g

Buckwheat Pancakes

Prep Time: 15 minutes

Cook Time: 10 minutes

Yield: 4 servings

Ingredients:

- 1 1/2 c. buckwheat flour
- 1/2 c. whole wheat flour
- 2 tsp. baking powder
- 1 tsp. baking soda
- 1/2 tsp. salt
- 3 T. molasses or honey
- 2 eggs, beaten
- 2 T. butter, melted
- 2 c. buttermilk

Directions:

Preheat a griddle or large skillet to medium-high heat. In a large bowl, combine dry ingredients (flours, baking powder, soda, and salt). In another bowl or measuring cup, whisk together molasses, eggs, butter, and buttermilk. Mix wet ingredients with dry until just incorporated. Allow the batter to sit for 10 minutes.

Ladle batter onto the griddle and cook, flipping when the top of the pancake is covered in bubbles. Serve warm.

Nutritional Information:

- Calories: 180

- Fat: 4.7g

- Cholesterol: 45.4mg

- Sodium: 387.8mg

- Potassium: 293.9mg

- Carbohydrates: 29.8g

- Dietary Fiber: 3.3g

- Sugars: 5.7g

- Protein: 7.1g

Apple Peanut Butter Breakfast Bars

Prep Time: 10 minutes

Cook Time: 12 minutes

Yield: 12 bars

Ingredients:

- 1/2 c. almonds
- 1/2 c. cashews
- 1 c. all-natural chunky peanut butter
- 1/2 c. golden flax seed meal
- 1/2 c. almond flour
- 1/4 c. honey
- 1 egg, beaten

Directions:

Preheat oven to 325°F. Line a square baking dish with parchment paper, allowing the edges of the parchment paper to extend over the edge of the pan. Blend almonds and cashews in a blender or food processor until finely chopped. Mix chopped nuts with all other ingredients in a large bowl. Pour contents into the parchment-lined pan and press evenly, being sure to get into all corners. Bake for 12 minutes, cooling completely before removing from the pan. Store in an airtight container in the refrigerator. The breakfast bars will keep for up to 2 weeks.

Nutritional Information:

- Calories: 270.9
- Fat: 20.5
- Cholesterol: 15.5mg
- Sodium: 42.7mg
- Potassium: 102.4mg
- Carbohydrates: 16g
- Dietary Fiber: 4.7g
- Sugars: 7.2g
- Protein: 10g

Black Bean Huevos Rancheros

Prep Time: 10 minutes

Cook Time: 25 minutes

Yield: 4 servings

Ingredients:

- 1 (14 oz.) can petite diced tomatoes
- 1/2 medium onion, diced
- 1 bunch cilantro, chopped
- 1 jalapeño pepper, diced
- juice of 1 lime
- 4 corn tortillas
- 4 eggs
- 1 (14 oz.) can seasoned black beans
- 1/2 c. shredded cheddar cheese
- kosher salt
- freshly ground pepper
- canola oil

Directions:

Make a simple pico de gallo by combining tomatoes, onion, cilantro, jalapeño, and lime juice. Season with salt to taste. Chill pico de gallo while preparing the rest of the meal. Brush a small skillet with canola oil and set over medium heat. In a small saucepan, warm black beans, smashing slightly. Warm each tortilla until lightly browned on each side, about 4 minutes. Fry eggs one at a time in the warm skillet to desired doneness.

To assemble: spread beans on top of each tortilla. Top with a fried egg, shredded cheese, and prepared pico de gallo. Season with salt and pepper to taste.

Nutritional Information:

- Calories: 271.3
- Fat: 11.4g
- Cholesterol: 203.9mg
- Sodium: 372.5mg
- Potassium: 389.8mg
- Carbohydrates: 29.8g
- Dietary Fiber: 8.5g
- Sugars: 4.2g
- Protein: 18.5g

Spinach and Mushroom Frittata

Prep Time: 15 minutes

Cook Time: 25 minutes

Yield: 6 servings

Ingredients:

- 2 slices thick-cut bacon
- 8 oz. sliced mushrooms
- 2 c. baby spinach, washed
- 1 medium onion, diced
- 8 eggs, beaten
- 1/4 c. milk
- 1/4 c. shredded Monterey jack cheese
- 1/2 tsp. kosher salt
- 1/4 tsp. freshly ground black pepper
- hot sauce

Directions:

Preheat oven to 425°F. Fry bacon in a large cast iron skillet until crisp. Cool on a plate lined with paper towels. Sauté mushrooms, spinach, and onions in the hot bacon grease until the spinach is wilted and the mushrooms are brown (about 4 minutes). Set aside to cool. In a large bowl, whisk together eggs, milk, cheese, salt, pepper, and hot sauce to taste. Crumble in bacon. Stir in cooled spinach, mushrooms, and onion. Pour mixture back into the cast iron skillet and cook over medium heat for 2 minutes. Transfer to the oven and bake for 15 minutes or until the top is golden brown. Serve warm or cold.

Nutritional Information:

- Calories: 156.1

- Fat: 10.1g

- Cholesterol: 257.4mg

- Sodium: 361.3mg

- Potassium: 177.1mg

- Carbohydrates: 3.5g

- Dietary Fiber: 0.8g

- Sugars: 1.2g

- Protein: 12.1g

Avocado and Egg Toast

Prep Time: 5 minutes

Cook Time: 5 minutes

Yield: 1 serving

Ingredients:

- ½ avocado
- 1 tsp. lemon juice
- 1 slice whole wheat bread, toasted
- 2 eggs
- kosher salt
- freshly ground black pepper

Directions:

Mash the avocado with salt, pepper, and lemon juice. Spread avocado generously over both slices of the toasted bread. Top each slice with 1 egg, prepared to taste (both fried and scrambled make great choices). Season with extra salt and pepper if desired.

Nutritional Information:

- Calories: 384.6
- Fat: 24.7g
- Cholesterol: 372mg

- Sodium: 743.4mg
- Potassium: 705.7mg
- Carbohydrates: 26.9g
- Dietary Fiber: 8.1g
- Sugars: 2.3g
- Protein: 17.2g

Eggs Florentine

Prep Time: 5 minutes

Cook Time: 25 minutes

Yield: 6 servings

Ingredients:

- 4 T. unsalted butter
- 2 cloves garlic, minced
- 4 c. baby spinach, washed
- 1/2 c. heavy cream
- 1/4 c. grated Parmesan cheese
- 1/8 tsp. cayenne pepper
- 1 T. lemon juice
- 6 fried eggs
- 3 whole wheat English muffins, split and toasted
- kosher salt
- freshly ground black pepper

Directions:

For the sauce: Melt butter in a large saucepan over medium heat. When the butter is melted, add garlic. Stir continually for 1 minute, taking care not to burn the garlic. Add spinach. Cook until the spinach has wilted and reduced (about 10 minutes), stirring occasionally. Add the cream and cook for 5 more minutes. Add the cheese, cayenne pepper, and lemon juice. Cook for another 5 minutes or until the spinach has reached the desired consistency.

To assemble: Top each English muffin half with creamed spinach and a fried egg. Salt and pepper to taste.

Nutritional Information:

- Calories: 303.1
- Fat: 21.8g
- Cholesterol: 237.2mg
- Sodium: 380.7mg
- Potassium: 167.5mg
- Carbohydrates: 16g
- Dietary Fiber: 2.9g
- Sugars: 3.3g
- Protein: 12.2g

Whole Wheat Waffles

Prep Time: 15 minutes

Cook Time: 10 minutes

Yield: 6 servings

Ingredients:

- 2 c. whole wheat flour
- 1 T. granulated sugar
- 2 tsp. baking powder
- 1 tsp. ground cinnamon
- 1/2 tsp. kosher salt
- 1 egg
- 2 c. whole milk
- 1/4 c. butter, melted

Directions:

Sift together flour, sugar, baking powder, and salt. In another bowl, whisk together egg, milk, and butter. Pour wet ingredients into flour mixture and fold in. Do not over mix. Allow batter to sit for 10 minutes before cooking. Ladle batter into a greased waffle maker and cook until slightly crisp.

Nutritional Information:

- Calories: 275.1
- Fat: 11.9g
- Cholesterol: 63.4mg
- Sodium: 375.4mg
- Potassium: 149.5mg
- Carbohydrates: 36.2g
- Dietary Fiber: 5.1g
- Sugars: 5.8g
- Protein: 9.1g

Breakfast Sausage Patties

Prep Time: 10 minutes

Cook Time: 75 minutes

Yield: 24 patties

Ingredients:

- 1 1/2 lb. ground turkey
- 1/2 lb. ground pork
- 1/2 c. grated onion
- 1 clove garlic, minced
- 1 T. extra virgin olive oil
- 2 tsp. kosher salt
- 1 tsp. freshly ground black pepper
- 1 tsp. fennel seed
- 1/2 tsp. dried sage
- 1/2 tsp. crushed thyme
- 1/2 tsp. crushed red pepper

Directions:

Combine turkey, pork, onion, garlic, and oil in a large bowl. In another bowl, mix salt, pepper, fennel seed, sage, thyme, and red pepper until combined. Shape sausage mixture into 1/4-inch patties. Refrigerate for 1 hour. Pan-fry over medium-high heat until brown, about 4 minutes per side. At this point, the sausage patties can be served hot or frozen between layers of parchment paper for up to three months.

Nutritional Information (per patty):

- Calories: 41.2
- Fat: 2.6g
- Cholesterol: 14.4mg
- Sodium: 174.3mg
- Potassium: 26.1mg
- Carbohydrates: 0.5g
- Dietary Fiber: 0.1g
- Sugars: 0g
- Protein: 4g

Baked Peach-Almond Oatmeal

Prep Time: 10 minutes

Cook Time: 45 minutes

Yield: 6 servings

Ingredients:

- 3 c. rolled oats
- 3/4 c. sliced almonds
- 1/4 c. brown sugar
- 1 tsp. kosher salt
- 1 tsp. baking powder
- 3 c. unsweetened vanilla almond milk
- 4 T. melted butter
- 2 eggs, beaten
- 2 tsp. vanilla extract
- 1 medium peach, chopped

Directions:

Preheat oven to 350°F. Grease a 9x13 baking dish with butter or non-stick cooking spray. In a large bowl, combine oats, almonds, salt, and baking powder. In another bowl, whisk together almond milk, butter, eggs, and vanilla extract. Mix all ingredients together.

Fold in chopped peaches and pour into prepared pan. Bake until the oatmeal is set and golden, about 45 minutes. Serve warm with a splash of cream or sprinkle of cinnamon if desired.

Nutritional Information:

- Calories: 370
- Fat: 19.6g
- Cholesterol: 75mg
- Sodium: 558mg
- Potassium: 494mg
- Carbohydrates: 40.2g
- Dietary Fiber: 6.5g
- Sugars: 9.4g
- Protein: 10.6g

Cinnamon Overnight Oats

Prep Time: 5 minutes

Chill Time: 8 hours

Yield: 4 servings

Ingredients:

- 1 1/4 c. rolled oats
- 1/2 c. plain yogurt
- 1 1/2 c. milk
- 2 T. ground flax seed
- 3 T. honey
- 2 T. ground cinnamon

Directions:

Mix all ingredients together in a large bowl. Divide equally between pint jars or another sealable container. Cover and refrigerate overnight.

Nutritional Information:

- Calories: 239
- Fat: 5g
- Cholesterol: 9mg
- Sodium: 68mg

- Potassium: 268mg
- Carbohydrates: 40.7g
- Dietary Fiber: 5.4g
- Sugars: 19.6g
- Protein: 8.9g

Chia Seed Pudding

Prep Time: 35 minutes

Chill Time: 8 hours

Yield: 4 servings

Ingredients:

- 1/3 c. chia seeds
- 1 1/2 c. unsweetened vanilla almond milk
- 2 T. pure maple syrup
- 1 tsp. vanilla extract

Directions:

Whisk together almond milk, syrup, and vanilla extract. Gently stir in chia seeds. Let stand for 30 minutes. Stir the pudding again to redistribute the seeds. Refrigerate overnight. Serve with berries or additional maple syrup if desired.

Nutritional Information:

- Calories: 115.4
- Fat: 4.7g
- Cholesterol: 0mg
- Sodium: 57.2mg
- Potassium: 157mg

- Carbohydrates: 13.5mg
- Dietary Fiber: 6.6g
- Sugars: 6.1g
- Protein: 4.1g

Drinks & Smoothies
Summertime Green Smoothie

Prep Time: 5 minutes

Yield: 2 smoothies

Ingredients:

- 1 peach, sliced
- 1 c. frozen strawberries
- 1/2 banana
- 1 c. raw baby spinach, washed
- 3/4 c. unsweetened almond milk
- 4-6 ice cubes

Directions:

Blend all ingredients until smooth. For a thicker texture, add 1/4 teaspoon xantham gum or up to 1/4 c. strawberry protein powder. Another option is to slice and freeze the banana before blending. If using frozen fruit, reduce the number of ice cubes by half.

Nutritional Information:

- Calories: 82.7
- Fat: 1.4g
- Cholesterol: 0mg

- Sodium: 74.8mg
- Potassium: 373.1mg
- Carbohydrates: 17.7g
- Dietary Fiber: 4.2g
- Sugars: 11.9g
- Protein: 1.9g

Berry-Oat Smoothie

Prep Time: 20 minutes

Yield: 1 large smoothie

Ingredients:

- 1/4 c. rolled oats
- 1/2 c. plain yogurt
- 1/2 c. unsweetened vanilla almond milk
- 1/2 c. frozen blueberries
- 1/2 c. frozen strawberries

Directions:

Mix oats, yogurt, and almond milk in the blender. Set aside for 15 minutes. Add berries and blend until smooth. For a thicker consistency, add 1/4 teaspoon xantham gum.

Nutritional Information:

- Calories: 230.2
- Fat: 7.3g
- Cholesterol: 15.9mg
- Sodium: 133.6mg
- Potassium: 422

- Carbohydrates: 35.9g
- Dietary Fiber: 6.1g
- Sugars: 16.2g
- Protein: 7.9g

Creamy Piña Colada Shake

Prep Time: 5 minutes

Yield: 1 smoothie

Ingredients:

- 1/2 c. unsweetened vanilla almond milk
- 1/2 c. coconut milk, frozen
- 1 scoop vanilla protein powder
- 1 oz. sugar-free vanilla flavoring
- 1/4 c. crushed pineapple
- 1/4 tsp. xantham gum

Directions:

Freeze coconut milk in ice cube trays at least two hours before preparing. Blend all ingredients until smooth. Up to 6 ice cubes can be added with the other ingredients if the coconut milk is not frozen, although the shake will not be as thick. Pineapple juice can be used in place of crushed pineapple for a smoother consistency.

Nutritional Information:

- Calories: 365.6
- Fat: 22.5g
- Cholesterol: 15mg
- Sodium: 260.3mg

- Potassium: 235mg
- Carbohydrates: 17g
- Dietary Fiber: 2g
- Sugars: 10.5g
- Protein: 24.5g

Chocolate Avocado Shake

Prep Time: 5 minutes

Yield: 2 smoothies

Ingredients:

- 1 medium avocado, sliced
- 1 banana, sliced and frozen
- 1 T. cocoa powder
- 1 scoop chocolate protein powder
- 1 1/2 c. unsweetened almond milk
- 6-8 ice cubes
- 2 tsp. mini chocolate chips (optional)

Directions:

Blend all ingredients until smooth. Top with chocolate chips, if desired. For a chocolate peanut butter variation, add 1/4 cup crunchy peanut butter with the original ingredients.

Nutritional Information:

- Calories: 287.4
- Fat: 17g
- Cholesterol: 7.5mg
- Sodium: 205.4mg

- Potassium: 789.7mg

- Carbohydrates: 23.9g

- Dietary Fiber: 9.6g

- Sugars: 7.9g

- Protein: 14.9g

Iced Green Tea

Prep Time: 5 minutes

Yield: 2 servings

Ingredients:

- 1 1/2 c. unsweetened vanilla almond milk
- 2 scoops vanilla protein powder
- 1 T. green tea powder
- 1 tsp. grated ginger root
- 2-3 T. honey
- mint leaves

Directions:

Blend almond milk, protein powder, green tea powder, and ginger root. Add honey to taste. Garnish with mint leaves and serve over ice.

Nutritional Information:

- Calories: 199.6
- Fat: 2.4g
- Cholesterol: 15mg
- Sodium: 273.5mg
- Potassium: 215.1mg

- Carbohydrates: 23.3g
- Dietary Fiber: 1.8g
- Sugars: 20g
- Protein: 22.8g

Soups & Stews
Tomato Bisque

Prep Time: 10 minutes

Cook Time: 20 minutes

Yield: 10 servings

Ingredients:

- 1 T. extra virgin olive oil
- 1/2 medium onion, diced
- 1 carrot, chopped
- 3 cloves garlic, minced
- 2 (28 oz.) cans whole tomatoes
- 1 (15 oz.) can cannellini beans, drained and rinsed
- 2 c. chicken stock
- 1/2 c. heavy cream
- 1 1/2 tsp. dried basil
- 1 tsp. kosher salt
- 1/2 tsp. freshly ground black pepper

Directions:

Heat oil in a large pot over medium heat. When the oil shimmers, add the onion and carrot. Cook, stirring often, until the onions are translucent (about 8 minutes). Add the minced garlic and cook for another minute, stirring constantly. Add tomatoes, beans, chicken stock, cream, basil, salt, and pepper. Puree with an immersion blender or in batches in a traditional blender.

Nutritional Information:

- Calories: 83
- Fat: 4g
- Cholesterol: 10mg
- Sodium: 514mg
- Potassium: 440.7mg
- Carbohydrates: 10.5g
- Dietary Fiber: 4.1g
- Sugars: 6g
- Protein: 3.2g

Better-for-You Minestrone

Prep Time: 15 minutes

Cook Time: 45 minutes

Yield: 8 servings

Ingredients:

- 1 c. pearl barley
- 1 T. extra virgin olive oil
- 2 cloves garlic, minced
- 1 medium onion, diced
- 2 large carrots, peeled and chopped
- 3 stalks celery, diced
- 4 c. chicken stock
- 1 (15 oz.) can petite diced tomatoes
- 2 c. chopped kale, stalks removed
- 1 (15 oz.) can kidney beans, drained and rinsed
- 1 (15 oz.) can navy beans, drained and rinsed
- 1 medium zucchini, diced
- 1 c. green beans, chopped
- 1 T. fresh lemon juice

- 1 tsp. dried rosemary, crushed
- 2 tsp. dried parsley
- 1/2 tsp. dried thyme
- 1 tsp. kosher salt
- 1/2 tsp. freshly ground black pepper
- 1/2 c. grated Parmesan cheese

Directions:

Heat a large pot over medium heat. Toast barley for 3-4 minutes. Set aside. Add oil to the pot. When the oil shimmers, add the onion, carrot, and celery. Cook, stirring often, until the onions are translucent (about 8 minutes). Add the minced garlic and cook for another minute, stirring constantly. Stir in barley, chicken stock, tomatoes and kale. Cover and heat until boiling. Reduce to a simmer and cook, covered, for 20 minutes.

Stir in beans, zucchini, green beans, lemon juice, and spices. Simmer for another 15 minutes. Serve with Parmesan cheese.

Nutritional Information:

- Calories: 238
- Fat: 7.48g
- Cholesterol: 11mg
- Sodium: 664mg
- Potassium: 725.1mg

- Carbohydrates: 34.4g
- Dietary Fiber: 7.1g
- Sugars: 5.6g
- Protein: 9.8g

5-Bean Chili

Prep Time: 15 minutes

Cook Time: 50 minutes

Yield: 8 servings

Ingredients:

- 1 T. extra virgin olive oil
- 1 medium onion, diced
- 1 cloves garlic, minced
- 1 large jalapeño, seeded and diced
- 1 bell pepper, seeded and diced
- 1 T. chile powder
- 2 tsp. ground cumin
- 1 tsp. ground coriander
- 1 tsp. kosher salt
- 1/2 tsp. dried oregano
- 1/2 tsp. black pepper
- 1 lb. lean ground beef
- 1 (28 oz.) can crushed tomatoes
- 1 c. vegetable stock

- 1 (15 oz.) can red kidney beans, drained and rinsed
- 1 (15 oz.) can black beans, drained and rinsed
- 1 (15 oz.) can pinto beans, drained and rinsed

Directions:

Heat oil in a large soup pot. When the oil is hot, sauté onion until translucent. Add garlic and cook for 1 minute, stirring constantly. Stir in jalapeño, bell pepper, and spices. Cook for 5 minutes. Add the ground beef and cook until brown, breaking up the meat with the edge of a spoon. Stir in tomatoes, vegetable stock, and beans. Reduce heat to maintain a low simmer for 35 minutes. Garnish with sour cream, grated cheese, or fresh cilantro leaves (if desired).

Nutritional Information:

- Calories: 289
- Fat: 11.3g
- Cholesterol: 50mg
- Sodium: 960.7mg
- Potassium: 702.6mg
- Carbohydrates: 26.1g
- Dietary Fiber: 8.4g
- Sugars: 6.3g
- Protein: 22.6g

Chicken Noodle Soup

Prep Time: 15 minutes

Cook Time: 35 minutes

Yield: 6 servings

Ingredients:

- 2 T. extra virgin olive oil
- 1 lb. boneless, skinless chicken breast, cubed
- 3 cloves garlic, minced
- 1 medium onion, diced
- 2 carrots, diced
- 3 stalks celery, diced
- 1 T. fresh thyme leaves
- 2 bay leaves
- 1 sprig rosemary
- 4 c. chicken stock
- 1/2 c. whole wheat angel hair pasta
- kosher salt

Directions:

Break pasta noodles in half and then in half again, making short, thin noodles. Set aside. This will keep the sugars down while still leaving plenty of noodles for each bowl. Heat oil in a large soup pot until simmering. Add chicken cubes and cook for 5 minutes, stirring often. Add garlic, onion, carrots, and celery. Cook for 4-5 minutes or until the onions are translucent, stirring regularly to keep the garlic from burning. Add thyme, bay leaves, rosemary, and chicken stock. Bring to a boil then add in pasta. Reduce the heat to maintain a steady simmer. Simmer 20 minutes. Salt to taste and serve. Remove bay leaves before serving.

Nutritional Information:

- Calories: 264
- Fat: 10.9g
- Cholesterol: 22mg
- Sodium: 454.8mg
- Potassium: 408mg
- Carbohydrates: 29.2g
- Dietary Fiber: 2.7g
- Sugars: 8.5g
- Protein: 12.2g

Butternut Squash and Granny Smith Apple Soup

Prep Time: 10 minutes

Cook Time: 35 minutes

Yield: 8 servings

Ingredients:

- 3 c. cubed butternut squash (fresh or frozen will work here)
- 3 medium apples, chopped
- 2 T. extra virgin olive oil, divided
- 1/2 tsp. kosher salt
- 1/4 tsp. freshly ground black pepper
- 1/2 c. diced onion
- 1/2 tsp. ground ginger
- 1/4 tsp. ground cinnamon
- 1.4 tsp. cayenne pepper (optional)
- 4 c. chicken stock

Directions:

Preheat oven to 400°F. Line a rimmed baking sheet with aluminum foil. Spread cubed squash and apples in a single layer on the sheet and toss with 1 tablespoon of olive oil. Sprinkle with salt and pepper. Roast for 20-25 minutes.

Heat the remaining oil in a large soup pot. Add onion when the oil is hot. Sauté onion for 7 minutes, or until the onion is translucent. Add ginger, cinnamon, and cayenne pepper (if using). Cook, stirring constantly, for 1 minute. Add chicken stock, squash, and apples to the pot. Bring to a boil. Puree with an immersion blender or in batches in a traditional blender. Check seasoning and serve.

Nutritional Information:

- Calories: 205.8
- Fat: 5.1g
- Cholesterol: 4mg
- Sodium: 320.2mg
- Potassium: 404mg
- Carbohydrates: 20.8g
- Dietary Fiber: 3g
- Sugars: 10.4g
- Protein: 3.2g

Hearty Lentil Stew

Prep Time: 10 minutes

Cook Time: 45 minutes

Yield: 8 servings

Ingredients:

- 4 T. extra virgin olive oil
- 1 medium onion, diced
- 1/2 c. diced celery
- 1 carrot, peeled and diced
- 3 cloves garlic, minced
- 1 tsp. ground coriander
- 1/2 tsp. ground cumin
- 1/2 tsp. ground thyme
- 1 lb. brown or green lentils, rinsed
- 1 (15 oz.) can diced tomatoes
- 2 qt. chicken stock
- 1 bay leaf
- 2 tsp. kosher salt
- 1 tsp. freshly ground black pepper
- 2 c. chopped spinach

Directions:

Heat olive oil in a large stock pot over medium heat. Add the onion, celery, and carrot and cook 8 minutes or until the onions are translucent. Add the garlic and cook, stirring constantly, for another minute. Add coriander, cumin, and thyme and cook until fragrant, about one minute. Pour in lentils, tomatoes, chicken stock, bay leaf, salt, and pepper. Bring to a boil. Reduce to a slow simmer and cook for 30 minutes. Add spinach and cook until the spinach is soft, about 5 more minutes. Remove bay leaf. Serve with fresh lemon juice or a splash of red wine vinegar. To make a vegan stew, replace chicken stock with vegetable stock or water.

Nutritional Information:

- Calories: 231
- Fat: 11.3g
- Cholesterol: 7.2mg
- Sodium: 1.1g
- Potassium: 517mg
- Carbohydrates: 24.2g
- Dietary Fiber: 3.1g
- Sugars: 6.4g
- Protein: 8.5g

Sausage and Chard Soup

Prep Time: 10 minutes

Cook Time: 40 minutes

Yield: 6 servings

Ingredients:

- 2 slices thick-cut bacon
- 1 lb. turkey sausage
- 1 medium onion, diced
- 2 c. white mushrooms, sliced
- 6 cloves garlic, minced
- 3 c. Swiss chard, washed and chopped
- 1 tsp. kosher salt
- 1/2 tsp. black pepper
- 4 c. chicken stock

Directions:

Cook bacon in a large pot over medium-high heat until crisp. Set aside on a plate lined with paper towels. Discard all but 1 tablespoon of the bacon grease. Brown the sausage in the rendered bacon fat and set aside. Add the onion mushrooms and sauté 8 minutes or until the onions are translucent. Add the chard and garlic to the pot and cook for 2-3 minutes or until the kale has started to wilt and the garlic is fragrant. Season with salt and pepper. Add chicken stock and simmer for 20 minutes. Return sausage to the pot and cook until heated through. Garnish with crumbled bacon.

Nutritional Information:

- Calories: 263
- Fat: 13.1g
- Cholesterol: 50.2mg
- Sodium: 1.2g
- Potassium: 485mg
- Carbohydrates: 17.5g
- Dietary Fiber: 1.2g
- Sugars: 3.7g
- Protein: 18.7g

Tortilla Soup

Prep Time: 10 minutes

Cook Time: 45 minutes

Yield: 6 servings

Ingredients:

- 3 T. extra virgin olive oil
- 2 c. diced onion
- 1 c. diced celery
- 2 carrots, diced
- 4 cloves garlic, minced
- 2 qt. chicken stock
- 1 (28-ounce) can crushed tomatoes
- 2-4 jalapeño peppers, chopped
- 1 tsp. ground cumin
- 1 tsp. ground coriander seed
- 1 tsp. kosher salt
- 1/2 tsp. black pepper
- 2 c. cooked chicken, chopped or shredded
- 1/2 c. chopped fresh cilantro leaves, optional
- 6-9 corn tortillas

Directions:

Heat 3 tablespoons of olive oil in a large pot or Dutch oven. Add the onions, celery, and carrots and cook over medium-low heat for 10 minutes, or until the onions start to brown. Add the garlic and cook for 30 seconds. Add the chicken stock, tomatoes with their puree, jalapeños, cumin, coriander, salt, pepper, and cilantro, if using. Cut the tortillas in strips and add to the soup. Bring to a boil, then lower the heat and simmer for 25 minutes. Add the chicken and cook for an additional 5 minutes. Serve topped with sliced avocado, sour cream, grated Cheddar cheese, or tortilla chips, if desired.

Nutritional Information:

- Calories: 472
- Fat: 27.1g
- Cholesterol: 41mg
- Sodium: 1g
- Potassium: 1g
- Carbohydrates: 28.1g
- Dietary Fiber: 6.8g
- Sugars: 9.2g
- Protein: 17.9g

Meaty Clam Chowder

Prep Time: 20 minutes

Cook Time: 25 minutes

Yield: 8 servings

Ingredients:

- 3 slices thick-cut bacon
- 1 medium onion, chopped
- 3 cloves garlic, minced
- 1 c. chicken stock
- 3 stalks celery, chopped
- 1 leek, washed and thinly sliced
- 1 bay leaf
- 1 lb. bay scallops, chopped
- 3 (10 oz.) cans fancy whole clams
- 1 (8 oz.) package cream cheese, softened and cubed
- 1 c. heavy cream

Directions:

Cook bacon until crisp in a large soup pot over medium heat. Set aside, reserving 2 tablespoons of bacon fat. Sauté onion and garlic in the rendered bacon fat until the onions are translucent, about 7 minutes. Add chicken stock, celery, and leek. Bring to a boil then add scallops and clams. Reduce heat to maintain a low simmer. Cook for 15 minutes. Remove bay leaf. Stir in cream cheese, letting the cheese melt completely before adding more. When the cheese is fully incorporated, add cream and salt to taste. Serve garnished with chopped bacon.

Nutritional Information:

- Calories: 337.3
- Fat: 24.1g
- Cholesterol: 133mg
- Sodium: 656.3mg
- Potassium: 412.1mg
- Carbohydrates: 9.5g
- Dietary Fiber: 1g
- Sugars: 1.5g
- Protein: 22.7g

Italian Wedding Soup

Prep Time: 10 minutes

Cook Time: 25 minutes

Yield: 8 servings

Ingredients:

- 2 T. extra virgin olive oil
- 1 medium onion, chopped
- 2 stalks celery, thinly sliced
- 2 carrots, peeled and chopped
- 2 qt. chicken stock
- 18 frozen, prepared turkey meatballs
- 2 c. chopped kale or chard
- 2 eggs, beaten
- 2 T. freshly grated Parmesan cheese

Directions:

Heat oil in a large pot over medium heat. Sauté onion, celery, and carrots in the oil until the onions are translucent, about 7 minutes. Add chicken stock, meatballs, and greens. Bring to a boil. Reduce heat to maintain a low simmer and cook for 15 minutes. While slowly stirring the soup, drizzle in beaten egg, breaking apart the egg strands with the spoon. Serve garnished with Parmesan cheese.

Nutritional Information:

- Calories: 148
- Fat: 9.2g
- Cholesterol: 69.4mg
- Sodium: 1.2g
- Potassium: 644.4mg
- Carbohydrates: 8.7g
- Dietary Fiber: 1.7g
- Sugars: 2.7g
- Protein: 9.4g

Main Dishes
Cucumber Tuna Salad

Prep Time: 10 minutes

Yield: 6 servings

Ingredients:

- 3 (7 oz.) cans albacore tuna in water
- 1 bunch green onions, thinly sliced
- 1 stalk celery, thinly sliced
- 2 dill pickle spears, diced
- 1/4 c. low-sugar mayonnaise
- 1/4 c. plain yogurt
- 3 cucumbers, peeled

Directions:

Slice cucumbers lengthwise and remove seeds. Drain tuna and break apart in a medium bowl. Mix in onions, celery, and pickle. In another small bowl, combine mayonnaise and yogurt. Fold into tuna mixture until well combined. Scoop into cucumber halves and serve.

Nutritional Information:

- Calories: 128
- Fat: 5.3g

- Cholesterol: 34mg
- Sodium: 365.1mg
- Potassium: 334mg
- Carbohydrates: 3.4g
- Dietary Fiber: 1g
- Sugars: 2.2g
- Protein: 16.8g

Avocado Chicken Salad

Prep Time: 10 minutes

Yield: 4 servings

Ingredients:

- 1 avocado
- 1 T. lime juice
- 1/2 tsp. kosher salt
- 1/2 tsp. garlic powder
- 1/4 tsp. freshly ground black pepper
- 1/4 c. chopped fresh cilantro
- 2 lb. leftover chicken, chopped
- 1/2 c. thinly sliced celery
- 1/4 c. diced onion
- 1/4 c. slivered almonds
- 2 T. low-sugar mayonnaise
- 2 T. plain yogurt

Directions:

Peel, seed, and smash the avocado with lime juice and spices. Mix with cilantro (fresh dill, basil, or parsley will work as substitutes if desired). Combine remaining ingredients in a large bowl with avocado mixture. Thin with 1-2 tablespoons cream if the mixture is too thick. Add more lime juice to taste.

Nutritional Information:

- Calories: 387
- Fat: 11.7g
- Cholesterol: 132.3mg
- Sodium: 432mg
- Potassium: 887.5mg
- Carbohydrates: 7.6g
- Dietary Fiber: 3.8g
- Sugars: 1.5g
- Protein: 24.9g

Spaghetti Squash with Meat Sauce

Prep Time: 15 minutes

Cook Time: 40 minutes

Yield: 4 servings

Ingredients:

- 1 large spaghetti squash
- 1 medium onion, diced
- 2 cloves garlic, minced
- 1 lb. ground beef
- 1 tsp. dried basil
- 1/2 tsp. dried oregano
- 1/2 tsp. red pepper flakes
- 1/2 tsp. kosher salt
- 1 (28-oz.) can whole, peeled tomatoes
- 1 T. red wine vinegar

Directions:

Preheat oven to 425°F. Microwave spaghetti squash whole for 5 minutes. When the squash is cool enough to handle, slice in half lengthwise and remove seeds. Place squash with the cut side up in a shallow roasting pan and sprinkle with salt. Roast for 20 minutes. Cool slightly and then remove squash strands with a fork.

While the squash roasts, prepare the sauce. Heat oil in a large pot over medium heat. Add the onion and cook 8 minutes or until translucent. Add the garlic and cook, stirring constantly, for another minute. Add the ground beef and brown for 7 minutes, breaking apart any large chunks with a spatula or spoon. Add the spices and tomatoes. Bring the mixture to a simmer, cooking for 30 minutes. Add vinegar before serving.

Nutritional Information:

- Calories: 420
- Fat: 24.5g
- Cholesterol: 98mg
- Sodium: 476.1mg
- Potassium: 247.3mg
- Carbohydrates: 11.6g
- Dietary Fiber: 2.1g
- Sugars: 12.7g
- Protein: 25.2g

Green Chile Pork

Prep Time: 30 minutes

Cook Time: 2 hours

Yield: 8 servings

Ingredients:

- 2 medium onions, chopped
- 1 lb. tomatillos, husked, rinsed, and quartered
- 3 jalapeño peppers, halved
- 2 cloves garlic, minced
- 4 T. oil, divided
- 2 lb. boneless pork shoulder, cut into 1-inch cubes
- 5 c. chicken stock
- 1 c. chopped cilantro leaves

Directions:

Preheat oven to 400°F. In a large bowl, toss the onions, tomatillos, jalapeños, and garlic with 1 tablespoon of the olive oil. Spread vegetables into a single layer on a baking sheet lined with foil. Roast until soft and starting to brown, about 20-30 minutes, stirring twice.

While the vegetables roast, add the remaining oil to a large, oven-safe pot over medium-high heat. Brown the pork, in batches, until well browned. Put all of the pork back in the pan and cover with chicken stock. Add the roasted vegetables to the pot, cover, and place in the oven. Cook until the pork is very tender, about 1 1/2 hours.

While pork is cooking, puree cilantro in a food processor with 2 tablespoons water. When pork is tender, remove from the oven and stir in the cilantro puree. Season with salt and pepper to taste. Serve over brown rice or with softened corn tortillas.

Nutritional Information:

- Calories: 301.7

- Fat: 15.3g

- Cholesterol: 73.4mg

- Sodium: 292mg

- Potassium: 804.7mg

- Carbohydrates: 13g

- Dietary Fiber: 13.1g

- Sugars: 6.6g

- Protein: 19.7g

Roasted Salmon with Lemon

Prep Time: 5 minutes

Cook Time: 25 minutes

Yield: 6 servings

Ingredients:

- 1 salmon whole-side fillet, skin on
- 2 T. lemon juice
- 1 bunch fresh dill, chopped
- 4 T. butter
- 2 T. white wine
- 1/2 tsp. kosher salt
- 1/4 tsp. freshly ground black pepper

Directions:

Allow salmon to come to room temperature before baking. Preheat oven to 425°F. Mix dill and lemon juice in a small bowl. Lay fillet skin-side down on a parchment-lined baking sheet and cover with lemon-dill mixture. Top with butter, white wine, salt, and pepper. Bake uncovered until the fish flakes easily with a fork, about 20-25 minutes.

Nutritional Information:

- Calories: 146.7
- Fat: 10.9g
- Cholesterol: 49.1mg
- Sodium: 237.3mg
- Potassium: 269.5mg
- Carbohydrates: 0.8g
- Dietary Fiber: 0.1g
- Sugars: 0.2g
- Protein: 10.3g

Broccoli and Beef Stir Fry

Prep Time: 5 minutes

Cook Time: 20 minutes

Yield: 4 servings

Ingredients:

- 1/2 c. chicken stock
- 2 T. soy sauce
- 1 T. Thai chili sauce
- 2 tsp. sesame oil
- 1 T. cornstarch
- 1 T. canola oil
- 1 lb. flank steak, thinly sliced
- 3 cloves garlic, minced
- 4 c. broccoli florets
- 1/4 c. water

Directions:

Mix together chicken stock, soy sauce, chili sauce, sesame oil, and cornstarch. Set aside. Heat oil in a large skillet over medium heat. Brown steak slices, stirring often, for 5 minutes. Add garlic and cook for an additional minute. Remove steak and garlic from the pan and set aside. Put broccoli and water in the pan, stirring to scrape up any bits left by the steak. Cover and cook for 7 minutes. Remove lid and stir in steak and sauce mixture. Stir to coat and cook for 4 more minutes. Serve over brown rice.

Nutritional Information:

- Calories: 245
- Fat: 11.2g
- Cholesterol: 70.3mg
- Sodium: 568.8mg
- Potassium: 544.2mg
- Carbohydrates: 5.4g
- Dietary Fiber: 1.2g
- Sugars: 1g
- Protein: 17.9g

Pork Tenderloin with Soy Sauce Marinade

Prep Time: 1 hour

Cook Time: 40 minutes

Yield: 6 servings

Ingredients:

- 1 1/2 lb. pork tenderloin
- 1 T. fresh ginger root, peeled and finely chopped
- 3 cloves garlic, minced
- 1/4 c. chopped green onions
- 3 T. soy sauce
- 2 T. red pepper flakes
- 1/4 c. rice wine vinegar
- 2 tsp. cornstarch, dissolved in cold water

Directions:

Marinate pork tenderloin in combination of chopped ginger, onion, garlic, soy sauce, red pepper flakes, and vinegar for 30 minutes or up to 6 hours. Preheat oven to 425°F. Remove pork from marinade, reserving remaining sauce. Bake tenderloin, uncovered, for 30-40 minutes or until the internal temperature reaches 160°F. While the tenderloin bakes, bring reserved marinade to a boil in a small saucepan. Add dissolved cornstarch.

Boil for 1 minute. Remove from heat. Allow pork to rest 10 minutes covered loosely with foil before slicing. Serve with sauce.

Nutritional Information:

- Calories: 177
- Fat: 4.1g
- Cholesterol: 83.6mg
- Sodium: 322mg
- Potassium: 540mg
- Carbohydrates: 2.6g
- Dietary Fiber: 0.6g
- Sugars: 0.5g
- Protein: 21.7g

White Spinach Pizza with Cauliflower Crust

Prep Time: 10 minutes

Cook Time: 25 minutes

Yield: 1 10-inch pizza

Ingredients:

- 1 head cauliflower, trimmed and chopped
- 2 eggs, beaten
- 2 c. shredded mozzarella cheese, divided
- 1/4 c. grated Parmesan cheese
- 2 tsp. Italian seasoning
- 3 T. extra virgin olive oil
- 1/2 c. shredded provolone cheese
- 3/4 c. whole milk ricotta cheese
- 3 cloves garlic, minced
- 1/4 c. thinly sliced red onion
- 1 c. baby spinach, washed

Directions:

To make the crust, pulse cauliflower florets in a food processor until they resemble rice. Microwave, covered loosely, for 5 minutes. Drain cauliflower in paper towel or cheesecloth, wringing out the towel to remove as much moisture as possible. Mix drained cauliflower with eggs, 1/2 cup of the mozzarella, Parmesan, and Italian seasoning. Press into a 10-inch round (or 10x15-inch rectangle) and bake at 425°F for 10-15 minutes. Brush crust with olive oil and top with remaining mozzarella, provolone, ricotta, garlic, red onion, and spinach. Bake for an additional 10 minutes or until the cheese is melted. This crust recipe will work with any toppings.

Nutritional Information (per serving):

– Calories: 350.3

– Fat: 25.6g

– Cholesterol: 116.7mg

– Sodium: 558.7mg

– Potassium: 415.8mg

– Carbohydrates: 9.3g

– Dietary Fiber: 2.8g

– Sugars: 0.8g

– Protein: 22.4g

Salmon Cakes with Homemade Tartar Sauce

Prep Time: 20 minutes

Cook Time: 15 minutes

Yield: 4 servings

Ingredients:

- 1/2 c. low-sugar mayonnaise
- 1 medium pickle, diced
- 1 T. chopped fresh chives
- 1 T. white wine vinegar
- 1 tsp. Dijon mustard
- 1/4 tsp. kosher salt
- 1 (15 oz.) can pink salmon
- 1/4 c. panko breadcrumbs
- 1/2 c. chopped onion
- 1 stalk celery, thinly sliced
- 2 eggs, beaten
- 3 T. canola oil

Directions:

Mix mayonnaise, pickle, chives, vinegar, and mustard until well combined. Add salt to taste. Chill sauce while preparing the salmon cakes. For the cakes, shred salmon with two forks in a large bowl. Add breadcrumbs, onion, celery, and eggs. Mix well. Form into 4-inch patties and chill for 15 minutes. While the salmon cakes are chilling, heat oil in a large cast iron skillet or griddle. Fry cakes for 5-7 minutes per side, or until golden brown. Serve with homemade tartar sauce or fresh lemon juice.

Nutritional Information:

- Calories: 510.8
- Fat: 41.7g
- Cholesterol: 184.2mg
- Sodium: 493.5mg
- Potassium: 534.6mg
- Carbohydrates: 5.6g
- Dietary Fiber: 0.7g
- Sugars: 0.8g
- Protein: 31g

BBQ Chicken

Prep Time: 5 minutes

Cook Time: 45 minutes

Yield: 6 servings

Ingredients:

- 1 whole chicken, in pieces
- 1/4 c. low-sugar barbecue sauce
- 1 tsp. kosher salt
- 1 tsp. garlic powder
- 1/4 tsp. freshly ground black pepper

Directions:

Preheat oven to 425°F. Arrange chicken pieces in a large roasting pan and brush with barbecue sauce. Season with salt, garlic powder, and pepper. Bake for 45 minutes. Let rest, covered, 10 minutes before slicing. Serve with extra barbecue sauce.

Nutritional Information:

- Calories: 181.6
- Fat: 4.3g
- Cholesterol: 103.4mg
- Sodium: 546.1mg

- Potassium: 384.7mg
- Carbohydrates: 1.4g
- Dietary Fiber: 0.1g
- Sugars: 0.1g
- Protein: 32.4g

Chicken Lettuce Wraps

Prep Time: 10 minutes

Cook Time: 15 minutes

Yield: 6 servings

Ingredients:

- 3 T. extra virgin olive oil, divided
- 1 T. fresh ginger root, minced
- 1 1/4 lb. chicken breast, cut into bite-size pieces
- 1 can sliced water chestnuts, drained
- 3/4 c. chopped mushrooms
- 4 T. rice wine vinegar
- 3 T. soy sauce
- 2 T. orange juice
- 1/2 tsp. garlic powder
- 1 c. shredded carrots
- 1/2 c. chopped green onion
- 1/3 c. sliced almonds, toasted

Directions:

Heat 1 tablespoon oil in a large skillet over medium heat. Add ginger, water chestnuts, mushrooms and chicken. Sauté until cooked through, about 7-10 minutes. Remove from heat. Once cooled, finely chop the entire mixture. Set aside. In a large bowl, whisk together remaining oil, vinegar, soy sauce, orange juice, and garlic. Add chicken mixture, carrot, green onion, and almonds to the sauce. Toss together. Serve with lettuce or over brown rice.

Nutritional Information:

- Calories: 256
- Fat: 15.1g
- Cholesterol: 60mg
- Sodium: 331.4mg
- Potassium: 391.7mg
- Carbohydrates: 6.2g
- Dietary Fiber: 1.3g
- Sugars: 1.6g
- Protein: 14.3g

Fried Brown Rice

Prep Time: 5 minutes

Cook Time: 15 minutes

Yield: 4 servings

Ingredients:

- 1 T. extra virgin olive oil
- 1 c. frozen mixed vegetables
- 2 c. cooked brown rice
- 1 egg, beaten
- 1 tsp. garlic powder
- 2 T. soy sauce
- 1/2 tsp. sesame oil
- 1 bunch green onions, thinly sliced

Directions:

Heat oil in a skillet over medium heat. Add mixed vegetables and sauté for 5 minutes. Add rice and cook until heated through. Pour egg into the rice and scramble, stirring regularly. Stir in soy sauce and sesame oil. Garnish with green onions.

Nutritional Information:

- Calories: 214
- Fat: 7.4g
- Cholesterol: 155mg
- Sodium: 303.7mg
- Potassium: 206mg
- Carbohydrates: 26.1g
- Dietary Fiber: 4.3g
- Sugars: 2.3g
- Protein: 6.9g

Black Bean and Sweet Potato Bowl with Lime Yogurt Drizzle

Prep Time: 20 minutes

Cook Time: 1 hour

Yield: 6 servings

Ingredients:

- 2 c. brown rice
- 3 c. water
- 2 T. butter
- 2 sweet potatoes, cubed
- 1 tsp. chili powder
- 1 tsp. garlic powder
- 2 (14 oz.) cans black beans
- 2 tsp. ground cumin
- 1 tsp. ground coriander
- 1 c. plain yogurt
- 1 c. cilantro leaves, roughly chopped
- 1 bunch green onions, diced
- 3 c. chopped romaine lettuce

- juice of 2 limes
- olive oil
- salt
- freshly ground black pepper

Directions:

Preheat oven to 400°F. Pour rice into an 8-inch square casserole dish. Cover with 3 cups boiling water, butter, and a pinch of salt. Stir to combine. Cover the rice with aluminum foil or a tight-fitting lid and bake for 1 hour. While the rice is baking, spread the sweet potato cubes on a sheet pan lined with foil. Drizzle with olive oil and season with chili powder, garlic, salt, and pepper. Bake the sweet potatoes alongside the rice for 20-25 minutes or until the sweet potatoes are soft.

While the potatoes and rice bake, bring the beans to a simmer in a small saucepan. Season beans with cumin, coriander, and salt to taste. To make the sauce, combine the yogurt, cilantro, and lime juice. Slowly drizzle olive oil into the sauce while whisking until the sauce is thin enough to pour easily. Chill the sauce until serving. To serve, fill the bottom of each bowl with lettuce. Top with rice, sweet potatoes, and black beans. Garnish with green onions and drizzle with cilantro-lime sauce.

Nutritional Information:

- Calories: 406
- Fat: 8.2g

- Cholesterol: 15.4mg
- Sodium: 800.1mg
- Potassium: 654.3mg
- Carbohydrates: 32.7g
- Dietary Fiber: 9.4g
- Sugars: 6.8g
- Protein: 11.2g

Braised Beans, Tomatoes, and Zucchini

Prep Time: 5 minutes

Cook Time: 15 minutes

Yield: 4 servings

Ingredients:

- 1 T. extra virgin olive oil
- 4 cloves garlic, minced
- 1/4 tsp. dried red pepper flakes
- 1/4 c. water
- 2 medium zucchini, diced
- 2 (14 oz.) cans navy beans, drained and rinsed
- 1 (14 oz.) can petite diced tomatoes
- 1/2 tsp. dried rosemary, crushed
- 1/2 tsp. kosher salt

Directions:

Heat olive oil in a large skillet with a lid. Cook garlic cloves and red pepper flakes briefly, being careful not to burn. Add water, zucchini, beans, and tomatoes. Cover and simmer for 15 minutes, stirring occasionally. Stir in rosemary and salt. More water can be added at this point if the stew is too thick. Serve warm.

Nutritional Information:

- Calories: 82.4
- Fat: 4.3g
- Cholesterol: 0mg
- Sodium: 415mg
- Potassium: 368mg
- Carbohydrates: 10.6g
- Dietary Fiber: 4.7g
- Sugars: 3.7g
- Protein: 2.7g

Sticky Coconut Chicken

Prep Time: 1 hour

Cook Time: 25 minutes

Yield: 4 servings

Ingredients:

- 8 boneless, skinless chicken thighs
- 1 c. canned coconut milk
- 1 T. minced fresh ginger
- 1 tsp. fresh ground pepper
- 1 tsp. red pepper flakes
- 3/4 c. rice wine vinegar
- 1/3 c. brown sugar
- 3 T. soy sauce

Directions:

Marinate chicken in coconut milk, ginger, pepper and red pepper flakes at least one hour or up to overnight. Grill on barbecue or broil. While the chicken is grilling, bring remaining ingredients to a boil over medium-high heat and cook until mixture is reduced and thickened, about 10 minutes. Once it starts getting really thick, remove from heat. Glaze both sides of chicken the last few minutes of grilling.

Nutritional Information:

- Calories: 228
- Fat: 12.1g
- Cholesterol: 0mg
- Sodium: 400.7mg
- Potassium: 298.1mg
- Carbohydrates: 23g
- Dietary Fiber: 3.6g
- Sugars: 15g
- Protein: 6.7g

Slow Cooker Recipes
Overnight Apple Cinnamon Oatmeal

Prep Time: 5 minutes

Cook Time: 8 hours

Yield: 8 servings

Ingredients:

- 2 c. steel cut oats
- 1 large apple, peeled and diced
- 1 tsp. kosher salt
- 1 T. ground cinnamon
- 2 T. brown sugar
- 2 T. butter
- 8 c. hot water

Directions:

Add all ingredients to a 6-qt. crockpot. Cover and cook on low for 8 hours. Serve with additional cinnamon to taste. Leftover oatmeal can be reheated in the microwave—simply add a splash of milk or cream after reheating to maintain the creamy texture.

Nutritional Information:

- Calories: 202
- Fat: 5.6g
- Cholesterol: 8.4mg
- Sodium: 319mg
- Potassium: 201.9mg
- Carbohydrates: 32.5g
- Dietary Fiber: 5.3g
- Sugars: 4.88g
- Protein: 6.7g

Homemade Plain Yogurt

Prep Time: 5 minutes

Cook Time: 10 hours

Yield: 8 cups yogurt

Ingredients:

- 1/2 gallon whole milk

- 1 (6 oz.) cup plain yogurt with active cultures

Directions:

Pour milk directly into the slow cooker and cook on high until the milk reaches 180°F (approximately 2 hours). The easiest way to monitor the temperature of the milk is with an instant-read thermometer. Once the milk reaches 180°F, turn off the slow cooker. Leave the lid on the slow cooker and allow the milk to come down to 110°F (about 3 hours).

In a small bowl, combine 1 cup of the warm milk with the plain yogurt. Whisk until the yogurt is thoroughly incorporated. Add the yogurt-milk mixture to the slow cooker by drizzling the mixture over the top of the warm milk. Do not stir or mix. Replace the slow cooker lid and wrap the cooker in a thick bath towel for insulation. Let rest for 8 hours or overnight. Homemade yogurt can be safely stored in the refrigerator for up to 2 weeks. For a thicker yogurt, strain yogurt through a cheesecloth-lined colander before serving.

Nutritional Information (per 1/2 c. serving):

- Calories: 117
- Fat: 4.02g
- Cholesterol: 13.4mg
- Sodium: 58.8mg
- Potassium: 169.9mg
- Carbohydrates: 16.2g
- Dietary Fiber: 0g
- Sugars: 16g
- Protein: 4.1g

Meat Lover's Breakfast Casserole

Prep Time: 30 minutes

Cook Time: 8 hours

Yield: 8 servings

Ingredients:

- 1/2 lb. pork breakfast sausage, cooked and crumbled
- 4 slices thick-cut bacon, cooked and chopped
- 2 medium baking potatoes, shredded and soaked
- 1 medium onion, diced
- 1 bell pepper (any color), diced
- 12 eggs, beaten
- 3/4 c. heavy cream
- 1 c. shredded cheddar cheese, divided
- 3 cloves garlic, minced
- 1 tsp. kosher salt
- 1/4 tsp. freshly ground black pepper

Directions:

Grease the slow cooker bowl with non-stick spray or butter. Whisk eggs, cream, salt, pepper, and half the cheese in a large bowl and set aside. Fill the bottom of the slow cooker with the shredded potatoes, pressing down on the potatoes to pack them lightly. Cover the top of the potatoes with the crumbled sausage and bacon. Add bell pepper and diced onion. Pour egg mixture over the top of the potatoes, meat, and vegetables. Top with remaining cheese. Cover and cook on low for 7-8 hours.

Nutritional Information:

- Calories: 529

- Fat: 35.6g

- Cholesterol: 965mg

- Sodium: 1.2g

- Potassium: 860mg

- Carbohydrates: 19.3g

- Dietary Fiber: 1.7g

- Sugars: 3.3g

- Protein: 19.7g

Homemade Pork and Beans

Prep Time: 5 minutes

Cook Time: 8 hours

Yield: 8 servings

Ingredients:

- 4 c. dried pinto beans
- 1 ham bone, split in half
- 1 tsp. salt
- 1 tsp. freshly ground pepper

Directions:

Sort beans and rinse in cool water. Pour the beans and ham bone into the bowl of a large crockpot and add enough cool water to cover by at least 2 inches. Cover and cook on low for 7-8 hours. If the bean sauce is too thick, more water can be added. Remove ham bones and add salt and pepper before serving.

This recipe can be prepared in 4 hours if the beans are soaked in cool water overnight. If you opt for this method, rinse the beans after soaking and cover with fresh water before cooking.

Nutritional Information:

- Calories: 336
- Fat: 1.2g

- Cholesterol: 0mg
- Sodium: 302mg
- Potassium: 1.3g
- Carbohydrates: 48.4g
- Dietary Fiber: 12g
- Sugars: 1.6g
- Protein: 16.6g

Pot Roast

Prep Time: 10 minutes

Cook Time: 8 hours

Yield: 8 servings

Ingredients:

- 4 lb. boneless chuck roast
- 1 (14 oz.) can petite diced tomatoes
- 4 carrots, peeled and roughly chopped
- 2 medium onions, quartered
- 4 cloves garlic, peeled
- 1 tsp. kosher salt
- freshly ground black pepper
- 2 bay leaves
- 1/4 c. water

Directions:

Place roast at the bottom of a large crockpot bowl. Cover roast with tomatoes, carrots, onions, and garlic. Season with salt, pepper, and bay leaves. Layer mushrooms, carrots, and onions on top of the roast. Tuck garlic around the edges and season with salt, pepper, and bay leaf. Add water and cover. Cook on low for 6-8 hours or until the roast falls apart.

Nutritional Information:

- Calories: 445
- Fat: 19.1g
- Cholesterol: 118mg
- Sodium: 546.3mg
- Potassium: 983mg
- Carbohydrates: 6.9g
- Dietary Fiber: 2.2g
- Sugars: 3.3g
- Protein: 61.4g

Garlic Roast Chicken

Prep Time: 10 minutes

Cook Time: 5 hours

Yield: 6 servings

Ingredients:

- 1 4lb. whole chicken
- 6 cloves garlic, peeled
- 1 tsp. garlic powder
- 1 tsp. kosher salt
- 1/2 tsp. freshly ground black pepper

Directions:

Remove giblets if included. Place the chicken breast-side up in the bowl of the crockpot. Arrange garlic cloves around the chicken, tucking them inside the legs and wings. Season with garlic powder, salt, and pepper. Cover and cook on low for 4-5 hours. For a crispy skin, broil the chicken for up to 5 minutes right before serving.

Nutritional Information:

- Calories: 349
- Fat: 6.9g
- Cholesterol: 185mg

- Sodium: 531mg
- Potassium: 738mg
- Carbohydrates: 1.4g
- Sugars: 0g
- Protein: 61.7g

Spicy Shredded Beef

Prep Time: 15 minutes

Cook Time: 10 hours

Yield: 10 servings

Ingredients:

- 5-6 lb. beef brisket
- 1 (7 oz.) can chipotle peppers in adobo sauce
- 1 (14 oz.) can petite diced tomatoes
- 4 cloves garlic, minced
- 1 medium onion, quartered
- 2 tsp. kosher salt
- 3 bay leaves
- 1/2 c. apple cider vinegar
- 2 c. water

Directions:

Place brisket at the bottom of a large slow cooker. Cover with chipotle peppers, tomatoes, garlic, and onion. Season with salt and arrange bay leaves on top. Pour vinegar and water around the brisket. Cover and cook on low for 8-10 hours. Serve shredded beef in enchiladas, tacos, or over grits.

Nutritional Information:

- Calories: 512
- Fat: 37.3g
- Cholesterol: 135mg
- Sodium: 3.5g
- Potassium: 866.7mg
- Carbohydrates: 3.9g
- Dietary Fiber: 1.1g
- Sugars: 1.8g
- Protein: 37.3g

Indian Butter Chicken

Prep Time: 10 minutes

Cook Time: 6-8 hours

Yield: 6 servings

Ingredients:

- 1 lb. boneless, skinless chicken meat (breast or thigh), cubed
- 1 (14 oz.) can garbanzo beans or chickpeas
- 1 small yellow onion, diced
- 4 cloves garlic, minced
- 1 T. curry powder
- 2 T. red curry paste
- 2 T. garam masala
- 1 tsp. turmeric
- 1 (4 oz.) can tomato paste
- 1 (14 oz.) can coconut milk
- 1 cup plain, low-fat yogurt
- 1/2 tsp. kosher salt
- freshly ground black pepper
- 2 T. butter
- 2 T. cilantro, chopped

Directions:

Season chicken chunks with salt and pepper, then set aside. Combine curry powder, curry paste, garam masala, turmeric, tomato paste, and coconut milk in a medium bowl. Grease the bowl of the slow cooker with cooking spray or butter. Layer chicken pieces, onion, and chickpeas in the greased bowl. Cover with the curry mixture. Top with butter, cover, and cook on low for 6-8 hours. Serve with fresh cilantro garnish over brown rice.

Nutritional Information:

- Calories: 266
- Fat: 9.34g
- Cholesterol: 71mg
- Sodium: 470.8mg
- Potassium: 868mg
- Carbohydrates: 23.3g
- Dietary Fiber: 7.7g
- Sugars: 8.7g
- Protein: 24g

Creamy Chicken Enchilada Soup

Prep Time: 10 minutes

Cook Time: 4 hours

Yield: 6 servings

Ingredients:

- 3 boneless, skinless chicken breasts
- 2 (14 oz.) cans black beans, drained and rinsed
- 1 medium onion, diced
- 2 cloves garlic, minced
- 1 (14 oz.) can diced tomatoes
- 1 (4 oz.) can diced green chiles
- 4 oz. cream cheese, cubed
- 1 T. cumin powder
- 1/2 tsp. kosher salt
- 1 c. green enchilada sauce
- 2 c. chicken broth

Directions:

Layer chicken, beans, onion, garlic, tomatoes, green chiles, and cream cheese in the bowl of a large slow cooker. Season the layered ingredients with cumin and salt before covering with enchilada sauce and broth. Cover and cook on high for 4 hours. Shred chicken before serving. Top with sour cream, shredded cheese, chopped cilantro, or diced avocado if desired.

Nutritional Information:

- Calories: 309
- Fat: 10.4g
- Cholesterol: 100mg
- Sodium: 1.5g
- Potassium: 954.8mg
- Carbohydrates: 12.8g
- Dietary Fiber: 7.6g
- Sugars: 6.9g
- Protein: 33.6g

White Bean Chili

Prep Time: 15 minutes

Cook Time: 8 hours

Yield: 8 servings

Ingredients:

- 2 lb. ground turkey
- 1 medium onion, diced
- 2 stalks celery, diced
- 1/2 c. diced bell pepper
- 1 (4 oz.) can diced green chile peppers
- 2 (14 oz.) cans navy beans, drained and rinsed
- 2 cloves garlic, minced
- 2 tsp. ground cumin
- 1 tsp. ground coriander
- 1 tsp. chili powder
- 1/2 tsp. dried oregano
- 4 c. chicken stock
- juice of 1 lime
- 1/2 c. chopped cilantro
- 1/2 c. shredded cheddar cheese

Directions:

Place turkey, onion, celery, bell pepper, green chile peppers, and navy beans in the bowl of a 6-qt. crockpot. Mix in garlic, cumin, coriander, chili powder, and dried oregano. Pour chicken stock over the top and cover the crockpot. Cook on low for 7-8 hours. Garnish with lime juice, cilantro, and cheese.

Nutritional Information:

- Calories: 277
- Fat: 13.9g
- Cholesterol: 95mg
- Sodium: 314mg
- Potassium: 553mg
- Carbohydrates: 11.7g
- Dietary Fiber: 2.5g
- Sugars: 4.3g
- Protein: 27.4g

Cheesy Grits

Prep Time: 5 minutes

Cook Time: 7 hours

Yield: 8 servings

Ingredients:

- 1 1/2 c. stone-ground grits
- 6 c. water
- 1 tsp. kosher salt
- 6 T. butter
- 1/2 c. heavy cream
- 1/2 c. shredded cheddar cheese
- freshly ground black pepper

Directions:

Spray the bowl of a large slow cooker with non-stick cooking spray. Mix grits, water, and salt in the greased bowl. Cover and cook on the lowest setting for 7 hours or overnight. Stir in butter and cream when the grits have finished cooking. More cream (or hot water) can be used if the grits are too thick. Serve topped with shredded cheese and black pepper.

Nutritional Information:

– Calories: 187.3

– Fat: 16.7g

– Cholesterol: 51.2mg

– Sodium: 367.9mg

– Potassium: 21.4mg

– Carbohydrates: 7.1g

– Dietary Fiber: 0.5g

– Sugars: 0.1g

– Protein: 2.8g

Brown Rice Pudding

Prep Time: 5 minutes

Cook Time: 4-5 hours

Yield: 8 servings

Ingredients:

- 1 c. brown rice
- 3 T. dark brown sugar
- 1 tsp. cinnamon
- 1 (14 oz.) can coconut milk
- 2 c. water
- 1 tsp. vanilla extract
- 1/2 c. raisins (optional)

Directions:

Grease the bowl of a slow cooker with butter or non-stick spray. Add rice, sugar, and cinnamon to the bowl. Stir to combine. Stir in coconut milk, water, vanilla, and raisins. Cover and cook on low for 4-5 hours, depending on desired consistency.

Nutritional Information:

– Calories: 78.4

– Fat: 2g

- Cholesterol: 0mg
- Sodium: 4.3mg
- Potassium: 93.3mg
- Carbohydrates: 15.1g
- Dietary Fiber: 0.9g
- Sugars: 7.1g
- Protein: 1g

Vegetables & Sides
Spinach Salad

Prep Time: 10 minutes

Cook Time: 20 minutes

Yield: 8 servings as a side

Ingredients:

- 8 oz. baby spinach, washed and dried
- 2 eggs
- 6 pieces thick-cut bacon
- 4 white mushrooms, sliced
- 1 small red onion, thinly sliced
- 1/4 c. pickled beets (recipe on page 117)
- 3 T. red wine vinegar
- 1/2 tsp. Dijon mustard
- 1 tsp. sugar
- 1/4 tsp. kosher salt
- freshly ground black pepper

Directions:

Place eggs in a large pot with a lid and cover with cold water. Cook, uncovered, on medium-high heat until boiling. Once the water boils, remove from heat and cover. Let the eggs sit for 12 minutes. Drain immediately and rinse in cold water. Peel the eggs when cool enough to handle. Chill in the refrigerator for at least two hours before assembling the salad.

Fry bacon in a heavy-bottomed skillet until crisp, reserving 4 tablespoons hot grease. Drain bacon on a plate lined with paper towels. When the bacon is cool, roughly chop and set aside. Return 1 tablespoon of the bacon grease to the pan along with the mushrooms and red onions. Sauté briefly, just until the onions start to turn translucent and the mushrooms are soft (around 5 minutes).

For the dressing: whisk together the remaining 3 tablespoons bacon grease with the vinegar, mustard, sugar, salt, and pepper to taste. To assemble the salad, fill a large bowl with the washed spinach. Top with hard-boiled egg slices, bacon crumbles, warm mushrooms, warm onions, and pickled beets. Dress lightly with hot vinaigrette and serve immediately.

Nutritional Information:

- Calories: 113

- Fat: 8.8g

- Cholesterol: 41mg

- Sodium: 226mg

- Potassium: 308.7mg

- Carbohydrates: 3.7g

- Dietary Fiber: 0.9g

- Sugars: 2g

- Protein: 4.9g

Spiced Butternut Squash

Prep Time: 15 minutes

Cook Time: 25 minutes

Yield: 4 servings

Ingredients:

- 1 large butternut squash, peeled, seeded, and cubed
- 3 T. extra virgin olive oil
- 1 T. brown sugar
- 1 tsp. ground cinnamon
- 1 tsp. kosher salt
- 1/2 tsp. freshly ground black pepper

Directions:

Preheat oven to 425°F. Line a sheet pan with foil and spray with non-stick cooking spray. Toss cubed squash in olive oil and spread in a single layer on the pan. Sprinkle with sugar, cinnamon, salt, and pepper. Bake for 25 minutes.

Nutritional Information:

- Calories: 132
- Fat: 10.6g
- Cholesterol: 0mg

- Sodium: 585mg
- Potassium: 255mg
- Carbohydrates: 11g
- Dietary Fiber: 1.8g
- Sugars: 3.7g
- Protein: 0.8g

Quick Pickled Beets

Prep Time: 10 minutes

Cook Time: 1 hour

Yield: 8 servings

Ingredients:

- 2 lbs. medium beets, peeled and rinsed
- 1 small red onion, thinly sliced
- 1 c. apple cider vinegar
- 1 c. water
- 1/4 c. granulated sugar
- 1 cinnamon stick
- 4 whole peppercorns
- 2 whole cloves

Directions:

Slice beets into wedges or rings and steam until tender (about 10 minutes). While the beets steam, heat vinegar, water, sugar, and spices to a low boil in a small saucepan. Add onion and simmer for 5 minutes. Pour spice mixture over beets and marinate for at least 30 minutes. For best flavor, marinate the beets for 2-3 days before serving. Beets and liquid can be refrigerated in a sealed container for up to 6 weeks.

Nutritional Information:

- Calories: 83
- Fat: 0.2g
- Cholesterol: 0mg
- Sodium: 90mg
- Potassium: 381mg
- Carbohydrates: 18.6g
- Dietary Fiber: 2.5g
- Sugars: 9.8mg
- Protein: 2g

Bacon Asparagus Bundles

Prep Time: 10 minutes

Cook Time: 20 minutes

Yield: 4 servings

Ingredients:

- 1 1/2 lb. asparagus spears, washed and trimmed (about 24 spears)
- 8 slices thick-cut bacon
- extra virgin olive oil
- 1 tsp. kosher salt
- 1/2 tsp. freshly ground black pepper

Directions:

Preheat oven to 400°F. Line a 9x13 casserole pan with foil and grease lightly. Toss asparagus spears in olive oil to coat. Divide asparagus into 8 equal groups (about 3 spears per bundle) and wrap each with a single slice of bacon. Tuck the bacon end into the bacon wrap. Each bundle can be secured with a toothpick if desired. Arrange asparagus bundles in a single layer in the casserole pan and season with salt and pepper. Bake for 15-20 minutes or until the bacon is crispy. Remove toothpicks before serving (if applicable).

Nutritional Information (per serving):

- Calories: 192.4
- Fat: 14.7g
- Cholesterol: 25mg
- Sodium: 622mg
- Potassium: 263.7mg
- Carbohydrate: 4.4g
- Dietary Fiber: 0.7g
- Sugars: 1.2g
- Protein: 10.2g

Balsamic-Glazed Brussels Sprouts

Prep Time: 5 minutes

Cook Time: 10 minutes

Yield: 4 servings

Ingredients:

- 1 lb. Brussels sprouts, washed and sliced in half
- 2 strips thick-cut bacon
- 1 medium onion, diced
- 1/4 c. balsamic vinegar
- 1/2 tsp. kosher salt
- 1/4 tsp. freshly ground black pepper

Directions:

Cook bacon in a large skillet over medium heat until crisp. Set aside on a plate lined with paper towels. Sauté Brussels sprouts and onion 3 minutes in 1 tablespoon reserved bacon fat. Add balsamic vinegar and cook until the vinegar has reduced, about 4 more minutes. Season with salt and pepper and serve warm.

Nutritional Information:

- Calories: 166g
- Fat: 4.4g
- Cholesterol: 10mg

- Sodium: 540mg
- Potassium: 547mg
- Carbohydrates: 13.2g
- Dietary Fiber: 4.9g
- Sugars: 3.7g
- Protein: 7.7g

Mashed Cauliflower "Potatoes"

Prep Time: 10 minutes

Cook Time: 30 minutes

Yield: 6 servings

Ingredients:

- 1 large head cauliflower
- 1 T. extra virgin olive oil
- 1/2 tsp. kosher salt
- 1/4 tsp. freshly ground black pepper
- 1/2 c. heavy cream
- 1/2 c. sour cream
- 2 T. unsalted butter
- 1/4 c. sharp cheddar cheese

Directions:

Remove outside leaves from cauliflower and quarter. Remove the core stem from each quarter. This will allow the cauliflower florets to separate. Wash and drain florets. Preheat oven to 400°F. Spread the cauliflower out on a greased cookie sheet. Toss with oil, salt, and pepper. Bake for 25-30 minutes. While the cauliflower is baking, heat cream, sour cream, and butter in a microwave-safe bowl. Combine cauliflower and cream mixture in a large bowl and puree with an immersion blender or in small batches in a traditional blender. More cream may be added if the puree is too dry. Serve with cheese and additional salt if desired.

Nutritional Information:

- Calories: 154

- Fat: 13.8g

- Cholesterol: 41mg

- Sodium: 308mg

- Potassium: 191.2mg

- Carbohydrate: 4.1g

- Protein: 4g

- Dietary Fiber: 0.9g

- Sugars: 1.1g

- Protein: 4g

Grilled Romaine Boats

Prep Time: 10 minutes

Cook Time: 5 minutes

Yield: 4 servings

Ingredients:

- 2 romaine hearts
- 2 T. balsamic vinegar
- 1 c. diced tomatoes
- 1/2 c. kalamata olives, pitted and sliced
- 1/4 c. feta cheese
- 2 T. grated parmesan cheese
- juice of 1 lemon
- olive oil
- salt
- freshly ground black pepper

Directions:

Heat a grill or grill pan to medium-low. Slice romaine hearts in half lengthwise, leaving the root end to hold the lettuce leaves together. Brush the cut ends of the romaine with olive oil and sprinkle with salt and pepper. Char the lettuce by grilling face down for two minutes. Arrange the grilled romaine halves on a plate and drizzle with balsamic vinegar and lemon juice. Top with tomatoes, olives, and cheese. Serve warm.

Nutritional Information:

- Calories: 87
- Fat: 7.5g
- Cholesterol: 9mg
- Sodium: 550mg
- Potassium: 133mg
- Carbohydrates: 3.5g
- Dietary Fiber: 1.1g
- Sugars: 1.7g
- Protein: 2.1g

Oven-Roasted Sweet Potatoes

Prep Time: 10 minutes

Cook Time: 20 minutes

Yield: 6 servings

Ingredients:

- 3 sweet potatoes, peeled and cubed
- 3 T. extra virgin olive oil
- 1 tsp. kosher salt
- 1/2 tsp. garlic powder
- 1/2 tsp. chili powder
- 1/4 tsp. freshly ground black pepper

Directions:

Preheat oven to 425°F. Line a large baking sheet with aluminum foil and spray with non-stick spray. Arrange sweet potatoes in a single layer on the baking sheet. Toss with olive oil and season with salt, pepper, chili powder, and garlic. Roast until the sweet potatoes brown and crisp at the edges, about 20 minutes.

Nutritional Information:

- Calories: 128
- Fat: 6.8g

- Cholesterol: 0mg
- Sodium: 437mg
- Potassium: 271.1mg
- Carbohydrates: 16g
- Dietary Fiber: 2.8g
- Sugars: 3.2g
- Protein: 1.3g

Garlicky Greens

Prep Time: 5 minutes

Cook Time: 15 minutes

Yield: 4 servings

Ingredients:

- 2 T. extra virgin olive oil
- 1 bunch kale or other leafy greens, washed and trimmed
- 3 cloves garlic, minced
- 1 c. chicken stock
- 1/2 tsp. kosher salt
- 1/4 tsp. freshly ground black pepper

Directions:

Chop kale leaves into 3-inch pieces. Heat oil in a large, lidded skillet over medium heat. Add kale and cook, stirring as needed, until the kale is wilted (about 3 minutes). Add the garlic and cook for 2 minutes more. Pour in the chicken stock and cook, covered, for 5 minutes. Remove the lid and cook for another 3 minutes. Serve with salt and pepper.

Nutritional Information:

– Calories: 99

– Fat: 7.1g

- Cholesterol: 0mg
- Sodium: 511mg
- Potassium: 343mg
- Carbohydrates: 8g
- Dietary Fiber: 1.1g
- Sugars: 0g
- Protein: 2.3g

Steamed Broccoli with Cheese Sauce

Prep Time: 5 minutes

Cook Time: 10 minutes

Yield: 4 servings

Ingredients:

- 2 T. butter
- 2 T. all-purpose flour
- 1/2 c. milk
- 1/2 c. chicken stock
- 1 c. shredded medium cheddar cheese
- 1/4 tsp. kosher salt
- 1/4 tsp. freshly ground black pepper
- 3 c. broccoli florets
- 1 T. butter
- 3 T. water

Directions:

Melt butter in a skillet over medium heat. Whisk in flour, cooking for one minute. Slowly add milk, whisking throughout. Once the milk is fully incorporated, slowly add chicken stock.

Cook, stirring often, for 5 minutes. Remove from heat and stir in shredded cheese, salt, and pepper.

Place broccoli florets, butter, and water in a microwave-safe bowl. Cover tightly with plastic wrap or a well-fitting plate. Microwave on high for 3 minutes. Check for doneness and microwave for an additional 1-1 1/2 minutes as needed. Season with salt and pepper to taste. Serve with warm cheese sauce.

Nutritional Information:

- Calories: 250
- Fat: 19.7g
- Cholesterol: 56mg
- Sodium: 465.9mg
- Potassium: 275.1mg
- Carbohydrates: 8.7g
- Dietary Fiber: 0.1g
- Sugars: 2.1g
- Protein: 10.6g

Easy Curried Lentils

Prep Time: 5 minutes

Cook Time: 25 minutes

Yield: 6 servings

Ingredients:

- 1 c. dried red lentils, rinsed
- 1 T. curry powder
- 1/2 tsp. kosher salt
- 2 c. water

Directions:

Sauté lentils, curry powder, and salt in a saucepan over medium heat until fragrant. Add water and heat to boiling. Cook, uncovered, for 25 minutes, adding more water if needed to keep the lentils covered. Drain lentils and serve.

Nutritional Information:

- Calories: 116
- Fat: 0.5g
- Cholesterol: 0mg
- Sodium: 199mg
- Potassium: 323.1mg

- Carbohydrates: 19.8g
- Dietary Fiber: 10.1g
- Sugars: 0.7g
- Protein: 8.4g

Three-Bean Salad

Prep Time: 15 minutes

Chill Time: 2 hours

Yield: 16 servings

Ingredients:

- 1 c. frozen petite corn
- 1 (15 oz.) can kidney beans
- 1 (15 oz.) can navy beans
- 1 (15 oz.) can black beans
- 1/2 c. red onion, diced
- 1 small bell pepper, diced
- 1 T. granulated sugar
- 1/2 c. extra virgin olive oil
- 1/4 c. red wine vinegar
- 1/2 tsp. kosher salt
- 1/4 tsp. freshly ground black pepper
- 1/4 c. chopped cilantro leaves

Directions:

Drain and rinse beans. Mix together in a large bowl. Add red onion and bell pepper. In another bowl, whisk together olive oil, vinegar, and sugar. Toss vinaigrette with bean mixture. Season with salt and pepper. Chill salad until ready to serve, at least two hours. Garnish with cilantro leaves and additional salt to taste.

Nutritional Information:

- Calories: 164.3
- Fat: 7.5g
- Cholesterol: 0mg
- Sodium: 169.9mg
- Potassium: 281.4mg
- Carbohydrates: 20g
- Dietary Fiber: 7g
- Sugars: 1.4g
- Protein: 6g

Green Beans with Caramelized Onions

Prep Time: 10 minutes

Cook Time: 35 minutes

Yield: 8 servings

Ingredients:

- 3 lb. green beans, ends trimmed
- 2 slices thick-cut bacon
- 3 T. butter
- 1 large red onion, sliced
- 1 clove garlic, minced
- 1/2 c. sliced almonds, toasted
- 1/2 tsp. kosher salt
- freshly ground black pepper

Directions:

Boil green beans in a large pot for 4 minutes. Drain beans and set aside. Fry bacon in a large skillet over medium-high heat. Remove crisp bacon to a plate lined with paper towels, reserving 2 tablespoons of bacon grease in the pan. Add butter and onions to the pan, cooking for 20-25 minutes. Add garlic and cook, stirring for 5 minutes. Add the cooked green beans and almonds. Season with salt and pepper and serve.

Nutritional Information:

- Calories: 141
- Fat: 8g
- Cholesterol: 13mg
- Sodium: 224mg
- Potassium: 436mg
- Carbohydrates: 15.2g
- Dietary Fiber: 6.9g
- Sugars: 3.4g
- Protein: 5.2g

Whole-Grain Greek Pasta Salad

Prep Time: 10 minutes

Cook Time: 15 minutes

Yield: 8 servings

Ingredients:

- 1 lb. whole wheat pasta
- 3 oz. grape tomatoes, halved
- 4 oz. feta cheese
- 3 oz. kalamata olives, halved
- 1 red bell pepper, diced
- 1/2 c. diced red onion
- 1 T. dried oregano
- 2 T. lemon juice
- 4 T. extra virgin olive oil
- 1/4 tsp. kosher salt
- 1/4 tsp. freshly ground black pepper

Directions:

Cook pasta according to box directions in a large pot of water. Drain pasta and set aside. While the pasta cools, whisk together oregano, lemon juice, olive oil, salt and pepper. Toss dressing with pasta. Stir in tomatoes, cheese, olives, bell pepper, and onion. Serve cold.

Nutritional Information:

- Calories: 211.8

- Fat: 13.5g

- Cholesterol: 12.6mg

- Sodium: 410mg

- Potassium: 87.4mg

- Carbohydrates: 18.7g

- Dietary Fiber: 2.2g

- Sugars: 1.6g

- Protein: 4.8g

Quick Coleslaw

Prep Time: 10 minutes

Yield: 6 cups

Ingredients:

- 1 T. extra virgin olive oil
- 1 T. rice wine vinegar
- 1/2 c. mayonnaise
- 1/4 c. sour cream
- 1 T. Dijon mustard
- 1 tsp. celery seeds
- 1/2 tsp. kosher salt
- 1/4 tsp. freshly ground black pepper
- 2 c. shredded green cabbage
- 2 c. broccoli slaw

Directions:

Whisk together olive oil, vinegar, mayonnaise, sour cream, and mustard. Fold in celery seeds, salt, and pepper. Toss with shredded cabbage and broccoli slaw. Serve cold.

Nutritional Information (per 1/2 cup):

- Calories: 71.3
- Fat: 5.5g
- Cholesterol: 2.1mg
- Sodium: 273.9mg
- Potassium: 193.7mg
- Carbohydrates: 4.1g
- Dietary Fiber: 0.7g
- Sugars: 0.8g
- Protein: 2.2g

Cauliflower Dressing

Prep Time: 20 minutes

Cook Time: 30 minutes

Yield: 8 servings

Ingredients:

- 2 medium heads cauliflower
- 1 T. extra virgin olive oil
- 1 large onion, diced
- 1 c. chopped mushrooms
- 2 cloves garlic, minced
- 4 stalks celery, thinly sliced
- 1/2 c. pecan pieces, toasted
- 2 T. chopped fresh sage
- 1 tsp. kosher salt
- 1/2 tsp. freshly ground black pepper
- 2 eggs, beaten
- 1/2 c. chicken stock

Directions:

Preheat the oven to 350°F. Trim stems and leaves from the cauliflower and roughly chop. Pulse cauliflower florets in a food processor in small batches until broken down to the size of rice. Set aside in a large bowl. Heat oil in a heavy-bottomed skillet over medium heat. Cook onions and mushrooms for 6-8 minutes, or until the onions are translucent. Add garlic and celery. Cook, stirring often, for 2 more minutes.

Add onion mixture to cauliflower and mix. Add sage, salt, and pepper. Stir in beaten eggs and chicken stock. Pour mixture into a greased casserole dish and bake for 25-30 minutes or until the dressing is golden brown and set.

Nutritional Information:

- Calories: 109.7
- Fat: 7.7g
- Cholesterol: 41mg
- Sodium: 355.6mg
- Potassium: 353.1mg
- Carbohydrates: 7.8g
- Dietary Fiber: 2.8g
- Sugars: 3g
- Protein: 4.4g

Desserts
Mexican Wedding Cookies

Prep Time: 15 minutes

Cook Time: 30 minutes

Yield: 2 1/2 dozen cookies

Ingredients:

- 1 c. butter
- 1/4 c. granulated sugar
- 1/2 tsp. kosher salt
- 2 tsp. vanilla
- 1 tsp. almond flavoring
- 1 c. whole wheat pastry flour
- 3/4 c. almond flour
- 1 c. finely chopped almonds
- 1/2 c. powdered sugar

Directions:

Preheat oven to 350°F. Cream butter, sugar, salt, vanilla, and almond flavoring. Combine with flours and pecans. Bake until just before the cookies start to brown, about 15 minutes. Once the cookies have cooled slightly, roll in powdered sugar.

Nutritional Information (per 2 cookies):

- Calories: 189.2
- Fat: 15.1g
- Cholesterol: 33mg
- Sodium: 174.8mg
- Potassium: 71.9mg
- Carbohydrates: 12.3g
- Dietary Fiber: 1.5g
- Sugars: 5.5g
- Protein: 2.2g

Pear Crumble

Prep Time: 10 minutes

Cook Time: 45 minutes

Yield: 8 servings

Ingredients:

- 4 large pears, chopped
- 1/4 c. granulated sugar
- 1 T. lemon juice
- 1 T. cornstarch
- 1 tsp. ground ginger
- 1 c. walnuts, chopped
- 2 c. rolled oats
- 1/2 c. all-purpose flour
- 2 T. brown sugar
- 1 tsp. ground cinnamon
- 1/4 c. butter, melted

Directions:

Preheat oven to 350°F. Mix pears, sugar, lemon juice, cornstarch, and ginger. Pour into a greased 9x13-inch casserole dish. In another bowl, mix walnuts, oats, flour, brown sugar, and cinnamon. Pour over pear mixture. Drizzle with melted butter and bake for 45 minutes.

Nutritional Information:

- Calories: 348.3
- Fat: 15.2g
- Cholesterol: 15.3mg
- Sodium: 47.2mg
- Potassium: 301.8mg
- Carbohydrates: 46.2g
- Dietary Fiber: 7.4g
- Sugars: 9.6g
- Protein: 9.3g

Grilled Peaches

Prep Time: 5 minutes

Cook Time: 20 minutes

Yield: 8 servings

Ingredients:

- 1/2 c. balsamic vinegar
- 1/2 c. honey
- 4 peaches, pits removed
- 1 T. extra virgin olive oil

Directions:

Combine vinegar and honey in a small saucepan over medium heat. Simmer until the mixture begins to thicken, about 10 minutes. Cut peaches in half and brush cut halves with olive oil and balsamic reduction. Grill, cut-side down for 7-8 minutes. Drizzle with remaining balsamic reduction.

Nutritional Information:

- Calories: 107.9
- Fat: 1.9g
- Cholesterol: 0mg
- Sodium: 5.8mg
- Potassium: 107.5mg

- Carbohydrates: 24.7g
- Dietary Fiber: 1g
- Sugars: 21.8g
- Protein: 0.4g

Cinnamon Apples

Prep Time: 5 minutes

Cook Time: 12 minutes

Yield: 4 servings

Ingredients:

- 2 T. butter
- 2 medium apples, cored and thinly sliced
- 1 tsp. ground cinnamon
- 1 T. maple syrup

Directions:

Melt butter in a skillet over medium heat. Add apples and cinnamon. Cook, stirring often, for 10 minutes. Add maple syrup and cook for an additional 2 minutes. Serve warm over ice cream or as standalone dessert.

Nutritional Information:

- Calories: 101.4
- Fat: 5.9g
- Cholesterol: 15.5mg
- Sodium: 41.5mg
- Potassium: 88.7mg

- Carbohydrates: 13.4g
- Dietary Fiber: 2g
- Sugars: 10.2g
- Protein: 0.2g

Super Soft Brownies

Prep Time: 10 minutes

Cook Time: 20 minutes

Yield: 1 dozen

Ingredients:

- 1 (15 oz.) can black beans, drained and rinsed
- 1/4 c. cocoa powder
- 1/2 c. quick oats
- 1 tsp. baking powder
- 1/2 tsp. kosher salt
- 1/4 c. canola oil
- 1 egg, beaten
- 1/4 c. honey
- 1 T. granulated sugar
- 1 T. vanilla extract
- 1/2 c. miniature chocolate chips

Directions:

Preheat oven to 350°F. Puree beans, cocoa powder, oats, baking powder, and salt in a food processor until smooth. In a separate bowl, whisk oil, egg, honey, sugar, and vanilla. Add bean mixture and stir until fully incorporated. Fold in chocolate chips. Bake in a greased 9x9 baking pan for 15-20 minutes. Let cool completely before serving.

Nutritional Information (per brownie):

- Calories: 173.4

- Fat: 8.9g

- Cholesterol: 31mg

- Sodium: 133.1mg

- Potassium: 93.1mg

- Carbohydrates: 21.5g

- Dietary Fiber: 2.9g

- Sugars: 12.4g

- Protein: 3.7g

Banana Bread Oatmeal Cookies

Prep Time: 10 minutes

Cook Time: 15 minutes

Yield: 18 cookies

Ingredients:

- 1 c. whole wheat flour
- 1 c. quick oats
- 1 tsp. baking powder
- 1 tsp. ground cinnamon
- 1/2 tsp. kosher salt
- 1 T. butter, melted and cooled slightly
- 1 ripe banana, smashed
- 1 egg, beaten
- 1 tsp. vanilla extract
- 1/2 c. brown sugar
- 1/2 c. chopped walnuts

Directions:

Preheat oven to 350°F. Combine flour, oats, baking powder, cinnamon, and salt in a large bowl. Set aside. In another bowl, mix together butter, banana, egg, vanilla, sugar, and walnuts. Stir dry ingredients into the banana mixture until combined. Be careful not to over mix. Drop in rounded tablespoons onto a parchment-lined baking sheet. Bake for 15 minutes.

Nutritional Information (per cookie):

- Calories: 92.8
- Fat: 3.6g
- Cholesterol: 12.1mg
- Sodium: 86.3mg
- Potassium: 72.8mg
- Carbohydrates: 15.4g
- Dietary Fiber: 1.7g
- Sugars: 6.4g
- Protein: 2.4g

Ginger Snaps

Prep Time: 15 minutes

Cook Time: 15 minutes

Yield: 18 cookies

Ingredients:

- 1/2 c. almond flour
- 1/2 c. oat flour
- 1 tsp. ground cinnamon
- 1 tsp. ground ginger
- 1/4 tsp. baking soda
- 1/4 tsp. kosher salt
- 1/4 tsp. ground cloves
- 1/ tsp. ground nutmeg
- 1/4 c. unsalted butter
- 1/4 c. granulated sugar
- 1 egg
- 1 tsp. vanilla extract
- 2 T. blackstrap molasses

Directions:

Preheat oven to 350°F. In a large bowl, sift together flours, cinnamon, ginger, soda, salt, cloves, and nutmeg. Set aside. In another bowl, cream butter and sugar until light and fluffy. Add egg, vanilla, and molasses. Gradually stir in dry ingredients until well combined. Wrap dough in plastic wrap and refrigerate or bake immediately. When ready to bake, use a cookie scoop to portion dough onto a parchment-lined baking sheet. Bake for 12-15 minutes.

Nutritional Information (per cookie):

- Calories: 78
- Fat: 4.2g
- Cholesterol: 17.2mg
- Sodium: 51mg
- Potassium: 85.9mg
- Carbohydrates: 8.8g
- Dietary Fiber: 0.7g
- Sugars: 2.9g
- Protein: 1.6g

Baked Vanilla Custard

Prep Time: 15 minutes

Cook Time: 1 hour

Yield: 6 servings

Ingredients:

- 1 c. heavy cream
- 1 c. unsweetened almond milk
- 4 eggs, beaten
- 1 T. granulated sugar
- 1 T. vanilla extract
- 1/2 tsp. ground nutmeg
- 1/2 tsp. ground cinnamon

Directions:

Preheat oven to 325°F. Heat cream and almond milk in a saucepan over medium heat until steaming. Do not let the cream mixture boil. Whisk eggs, sugar, and vanilla extract in a large bowl. Slowly ladle the hot cream into the egg mixture while continuing to whisk. Once the eggs are heated through, stir in the remainder of the cream mixture. Pour mixture into a casserole dish. Top with nutmeg and cinnamon. Place casserole dish in a larger baking dish on the middle rack of the preheated oven. Pour hot water in the larger dish. Bake for 1 hour. Serve warm or chilled.

Nutritional Information:

- Calories: 109
- Fat: 7.9g
- Cholesterol: 27.1mg
- Sodium: 70mg
- Potassium: 76.4mg
- Carbohydrates: 5.2g
- Dietary Fiber: 0.3g
- Sugars: 4.8g
- Protein: 3g

Chocolate Pots de Crème

Prep Time: 20 minutes

Cook Time: 30 minutes

Yield: 4 servings

Ingredients:

- 1 c. half-and-half
- 1/4 c. brewed coffee
- 1/4 c. semisweet chocolate chips
- 1 T. cocoa powder
- 1/4 c. granulated sugar
- 3 egg yolks
- 1 tsp. vanilla extract

Directions:

Preheat oven to 300°F. Heat half-and-half and coffee in a saucepan over medium heat until steaming. Remove from heat and stir in chocolate chips and cocoa powder. While the mixture cools, whisk together sugar, egg yolks, and vanilla. Gradually ladle chocolate mixture into the egg yolks until the yolk mixture is warm. Stir egg mixture into remaining chocolate and mix well. Divide mixture among 4 ramekins or custard cups and bake for 30 minutes. Chill, covered with plastic wrap, for at least 3 hours before serving.

Nutritional Information:

- Calories: 243.8
- Fat: 14.4g
- Cholesterol: 162.2mg
- Sodium: 30.9mg
- Potassium: 123.6mg
- Carbohydrates: 25.2g
- Dietary Fiber: 0.5g
- Sugars: 23.2g
- Protein: 3.9g

Melon Sorbet

Prep Time: 10 minutes

Chill Time: 8 hours

Yield: 8 servings

Ingredients:

- 1 c. cubed or balled cantaloupe
- 1 c. cubed or balled honeydew melon
- 1 T. light corn syrup
- 1 tsp. lime juice

Directions:

Freeze cubed cantaloupe and honeydew overnight. Pulse frozen melon in a food processor until pureed. Add corn syrup and lime juice and puree until smooth. More water can be added to reach the desired consistency.

Nutritional Information:

- Calories: 23
- Fat: 0.1g
- Cholesterol: 0mg
- Sodium: 9mg
- Potassium: 119mg

- Carbohydrates: 5.9g
- Dietary Fiber: 0.4g
- Sugars: 5.5g
- Protein: 0.3g

Tart Lemon Sorbet

Prep Time: 15 minutes

Chill Time: 2 hours

Yield: 8 servings

Ingredients:

- 2 c. water
- 2 c. fresh lemon juice
- 1 c. granulated sugar
- 2 T. grated lemon zest

Directions:

Combine water, juice, and sugar in a saucepan over medium heat. Boil for 2 minutes or until the sugar has dissolved completely. Remove from heat and chill before transferring to the ice cream maker. Add lemon zest and churn according to your ice cream maker's directions. Freeze at least 1 hour before serving. Garnish with mint leaves or fresh raspberries.

Nutritional Information:

- Calories: 111.2
- Fat: 0g
- Cholesterol: 0mg
- Sodium: 0mg

- Potassium: 0.7mg
- Carbohydrates: 30.5g
- Dietary Fiber: 0.4g
- Sugars: 26.5g
- Protein: 0.3g

Chocolate Cherry Frozen Yogurt

Prep Time: 5 minutes

Chill Time: 1 1/2 hours

Yield: 8 servings

Ingredients:

- 2 c. plain yogurt
- 2 packets stevia
- 1 tsp. vanilla extract
- 2 drops red food coloring (optional)
- 1/2 c. pitted cherries, chopped
- 3 T. miniature chocolate chips

Directions:

Mix yogurt, stevia, and vanilla. Churn according to your ice cream maker's directions. When the frozen yogurt is almost finished churning, add cherries and chocolate chips. Freeze yogurt in a covered container for at least an hour before serving.

Nutritional Information:

- Calories: 70.8
- Fat: 3.5g
- Cholesterol: 8mg

- Sodium: 28.2mg
- Potassium: 115.8mg
- Carbohydrates: 7.9g
- Dietary Fiber: 0.2g
- Sugars: 7.2g
- Protein: 2.2g

Cheesecake Ice Cream

Prep Time: 30 minutes

Chill Time: 2 hours

Yield: 8 servings

Ingredients:

- 1 (8 oz.) package cream cheese, softened
- 1/2 c. granulated sugar
- 2 T. corn syrup
- 1 c. heavy cream
- 1 c. low-fat buttermilk

Directions:

Blend cream cheese and sugar until soft and creamy. Add in corn syrup, cream, and buttermilk. Churn according to your ice cream maker's instructions. Transfer to a freezer-safe container and freeze for at least 2 hours before serving. Top with fresh strawberries, caramel sauce, or you other favorite cheesecake topping.

Nutritional Information:

- Calories: 274.2
- Fat: 21.1g
- Cholesterol: 73mg

- Sodium: 133.4mg
- Potassium: 107.8mg
- Carbohydrates: 19.9g
- Dietary Fiber: 0g
- Sugars: 18.9g
- Protein: 3.7g

Berries and Cream

Prep Time: 10 minutes

Yield: 4 servings

Ingredients:

- 1/2 c. heavy whipping cream
- 1 T. confectioner's sugar
- 1 tsp. vanilla extract
- 1/2 c. fresh raspberries
- 1/2 c. fresh blueberries
- 1/2 c. fresh blackberries
- 1 tsp. granulated sugar

Directions:

Toss berries and granulated sugar in a large bowl. Set aside. Place a metal bowl in the freezer for 15 minutes before whipping cream. Beat cream and confectioner's sugar in the cold bowl until stiff peaks form. Fold in vanilla. Serve immediately.

Nutritional Information:

– Calories: 141.5
– Fat: 11.2g
– Cholesterol: 40.8mg

- Sodium: 12.4mg
- Potassium: 97.1mg
- Carbohydrates: 10.5g
- Dietary Fiber: 2.5g
- Sugars: 6.2g
- Protein: 1g

Snacks
Avocado Bean Dip

Prep Time: 10 minutes

Chill Time: 1 hour

Yield: 10 servings

Ingredients:

- 3 large avocados, diced
- 2 medium tomatoes, seeded and diced
- 1 c. chopped red bell pepper
- 1 (15 oz.) can black beans, drained and rinsed
- 1 c. petite white corn
- 1 packet dry Italian dressing mix
- 6 T. lime juice
- 1/2 tsp. garlic powder
- 1/4 tsp. kosher salt
- 1/4 tsp. freshly ground black pepper

Directions:

Combine all ingredients in a large bowl. Chill at least 1 hour before serving. Serve with tortilla chips or as garnish on tacos, enchiladas, and more.

Nutritional Information:

- Calories: 154.6
- Fat: 8.9g
- Cholesterol: 0.5mg
- Sodium: 244.2mg
- Potassium: 368mg
- Carbohydrates: 16.4g
- Dietary Fiber: 7g
- Sugars: 1.5g
- Protein: 4.4g

Spiced Pecans

Prep Time: 5 minutes

Cook Time: 25 minutes

Yield: 8 servings

Ingredients:

- 4 T. butter
- 4 c. raw pecan halves
- 1 egg white
- 1 tsp. kosher salt
- 1 tsp. smoked paprika
- 1 tsp. ground ginger
- 1/2 tsp. ground cinnamon
- 1/2 tsp. freshly ground black pepper
- 1/4 tsp. cayenne pepper (optional)

Directions:

Preheat oven to 300°F. Melt butter in a large pan over medium heat. Add pecans and cook, stirring occasionally, for 5 minutes. While the pecans are cooking, whisk egg white until foamy. Stir in salt, paprika, ginger, cinnamon, and peppers. Fold the egg white mixture in with the pecans and butter. Spread nuts in a single layer on a parchment-lined baking sheet and bake for 20 minutes.

Nutritional Information:

– Calories: 428.6

– Fat: 44.7g

– Cholesterol: 15.5mg

– Sodium: 247.9mg

– Potassium: 235.9mg

– Carbohydrates: 8.1g

– Dietary Fiber: 5.4g

– Sugars: 2.2g

– Protein: 5.5g

Coconut Protein Bites

Prep Time: 20 minutes

Yield: 40 bites

Ingredients:

- 2 c. toasted almonds
- 2 c. shredded unsweetened coconut
- 1/2 c. flax seeds
- 2/3 c. coconut oil
- 1 c. almond butter
- 1 c. rolled oats
- 1/2 c. mini chocolate chips

Directions:

Pulse almonds, coconut, and flax seeds in a food processor until well chopped. Whisk coconut oil and almond butter together in a large bowl. Add in coconut mixture and mix until combined. Fold in oats and chocolate chips.

Scoop the mixture 1 tablespoon at a time and roll into packed balls. Chilling the mixture before rolling will make the process easier. Store in the refrigerator for up to 2 weeks.

Nutritional Information (per 2-bite serving):

- Calories: 343
- Fat: 31g
- Cholesterol: 0mg
- Sodium: 5.7mg
- Potassium: 227.6mg
- Carbohydrates: 15.8g
- Dietary Fiber: 5.8g
- Sugars: 4.9g
- Protein: 6.8g

Traditional Hummus

Prep Time: 5 minutes

Yield: 2 cups

Ingredients:

- 1 (15 oz.) can chickpeas, drained and rinsed
- 1/4 c. tahini
- 1/4 c. extra virgin olive oil
- 2 tsp. paprika
- 1 tsp. garlic powder
- 1 tsp. ground cumin
- 2 T. lemon juice

Directions:

Puree all ingredients in a food processor. Add water or additional oil to reach the desired consistency. Season with salt or additional lemon juice to taste.

Nutritional Information (per 1/4 cup serving):

- Calories: 181.2
- Fat: 11.8g
- Cholesterol: 0mg
- Sodium: 188.8mg

- Potassium: 162.4mg
- Carbohydrates: 16.3g
- Dietary Fiber: 3.6g
- Sugars: 0.3g
- Protein: 4.5g

Spinach Artichoke Dip

Prep Time: 15 minutes

Chill Time: 2 hours

Yield: 10-12 servings

Ingredients:

- 1 (4 oz.) package cream cheese
- 1 c. mayonnaise
- 1/2 c. plain Greek yogurt
- 6 marinated artichoke hearts, chopped
- 2 cloves garlic, minced
- 1 (10 oz.) package frozen spinach, thawed and drained
- 1 c. grated Parmesan cheese

Directions:

Beat cream cheese with a handheld mixer until smooth and fluffy (about 3 minutes). Mix in mayonnaise and yogurt until evenly combined. Stir in artichoke hearts, garlic, spinach, and cheese. Chill at least 2 hours before serving.

Nutritional Information:

- Calories: 266.1
- Fat: 26.8g

- Cholesterol: 36.3mg
- Sodium: 390mg
- Potassium: 94.3mg
- Carbohydrates: 3.6g
- Dietary Fiber: 0.7g
- Sugars: 0.8g
- Protein: 6.9g

Caramelized Onion Dip

Prep Time: 40 minutes

Chill Time: 2 hours

Yield: 8-10 servings

Ingredients:

- 3 T. butter
- 2 large yellow onions, thinly sliced
- 1 tsp. onion powder
- 1/2 tsp. garlic powder
- 1/2 tsp. kosher salt
- 1 (8 oz.) package cream cheese, softened
- 1/2 c. sour cream
- 1/2 c. plain Greek yogurt

Directions:

Melt butter in a large skillet over medium heat. Add onions and reduce the heat to medium-low. Cook, stirring occasionally, until the onions are golden brown (about 30 minutes). Remove from heat and season with onion powder, garlic powder, and salt. While the onions cool, beat cream cheese with sour cream and yogurt until smooth. Fold in onions. Chill at least 2 hours before serving.

Nutritional Information:

- Calories: 148
- Fat: 13.4g
- Cholesterol: 35mg
- Sodium: 263.9mg
- Potassium: 96.4mg
- Carbohydrates: 3.7g
- Dietary Fiber: 0.3g
- Sugars: 2g
- Protein: 3.5g

Spiced Edamame

Prep Time: 5 minutes

Cook Time: 10 minutes

Yield: 4 servings

Ingredients:

- 1 (1 lb.) bag frozen edamame in the pod
- 1 tsp. kosher salt
- 1 tsp. garlic powder
- 1 tsp. chile powder

Directions:

In a small bowl, whisk together spices. Set aside. Bring a pot of salted water to a rolling boil. Boil edamame for 8 minutes. Drain edamame and toss with spice mixture. Serve warm.

Nutritional Information:

- Calories: 143
- Fat: 5.9g
- Cholesterol: 0mg
- Sodium: 588.7mg
- Potassium: 510mg
- Carbohydrates: 12.3g
- Dietary Fiber: 6g
- Sugars: 2.5g
- Protein: 12.5g

Oven Beef Jerky

Prep Time: 2 hours

Cook Time: 5 hours

Yield: 2 lbs. jerky

Ingredients:

- 3 lb. flank steak or brisket, trimmed of fat
- 1/2 c. soy sauce
- 2 T. sesame oil
- 2 T. canola oil
- 1 T. Thai chile sauce
- 3 cloves garlic, minced
- 1 T. grated fresh ginger
- 1 tsp. coarse black pepper

Directions:

Slice meat against the grain into 1/4-inch strips. Meat that has been partially frozen (1-2 hours in the freezer) will be easier to slice evenly. In a large zip-top bag, combine remaining ingredients. Add the meat strips and turn to coat with marinade. Refrigerate for 2-8 hours, turning twice.

Remove meat from refrigerator to come to room temperature while the oven preheats. Heat oven to 170°F. Line 2 large baking pans with foil. Place cooling racks on the pans and spray racks with non-stick cooking spray. Remove meat from the marinade and arrange strips on the racks. Bake for 4-5 hours, checking every 30 minutes after 3 hours. Turn off the oven and allow jerky to cool completely in the oven before removing to an airtight container.

Nutritional Information (per 1/8 pound):

- Calories: 154
- Fat: 7.7g
- Cholesterol: 51.1mg
- Sodium: 346.2mg
- Potassium: 327.8mg
- Carbohydrates: 1g
- Dietary Fiber: 0.2g
- Sugars: 0.2g
- Protein: 19g

Curried Deviled Eggs

Prep Time: 15 minutes

Cook Time: 12 minutes

Yield: 24 deviled eggs

Ingredients:

- 12 raw eggs
- 1/4 c. mayonnaise
- 2 T. plain Greek yogurt
- 1 tsp. yellow mustard
- 2 tsp. white vinegar
- 1 tsp. curry powder
- 1/4 tsp. cayenne pepper (optional)

Directions:

Place eggs in a large pot cover with cold at least one inch of cool water. Cook, uncovered, on medium-high heat until the water reaches a roiling boil. Once the water boils, remove from heat and cover with a tight-fitting lid. Set a timer for 12 minutes. After the timer rings, drain the eggs and rinse in cold water. Peel the eggs when cool enough to handle. For easier-to-peel eggs, use eggs that are a week or more old.

While the eggs cook, combine mayonnaise, yogurt, mustard, vinegar, and spices. Slice eggs in half lengthwise and scoop yolks into a small bowl. Mix yolks with the mayonnaise mixture until smooth. Smashing the yolks slightly before mixing will lead to a smoother mix. If the yolk mixture is too dry, add additional mayonnaise or mustard until the desired texture is achieved.

With a spoon or small cookie scoop, fill the hollow of each egg white with a generous scoop of yolk mixture. Garnish with smoked paprika or chopped basil if desired. Serve immediately or cover with plastic wrap and chill until serving.

Nutritional Information:

- Calories: 31.3
- Fat: 1g
- Cholesterol: 1.3mg
- Sodium: 66mg
- Potassium: 62.3mg
- Carbohydrates: 1.2g
- Dietary Fiber: 0.1g
- Sugars: 0.6g
- Protein: 3.7g

Pantry Staples
Whole Grain Bread

Prep Time: 1 hour

Cook Time: 35 minutes

Yield: 2 loaves

Ingredients:

- 2 1/2 c. warm water
- 1 T. instant yeast
- 3 T. coconut oil
- 3 T. honey
- 1 T. kosher salt
- 1 c. quick oats
- 5 1/2-6 c. whole wheat flour

Directions:

Combine water and yeast in a small bowl. Set aside for the yeast to bloom, 2-3 minutes. In the bowl of a mixer with a dough hook attachment, combine oil, honey, salt, oats, one cup of flour, and the yeast mixture. Stir until combined. Let rest for 10 minutes. With the mixer on the lowest setting, add flour one cup at a time until the dough pulls away from the bowl and begins to climb up the dough hook. Knead for 7 minutes. Cover the bowl and let rest for 30 minutes.

Transfer the dough to a lightly greased counter. Divide in half and shape each half into a loaf the length and width of your bred pans. Place in greased pans, cover with lightly greased plastic wrap, and let rise in a warm place for about 30 minutes. After the dough has crowned one inch above the rim of the pan, place pans on the middle rack of a cold oven. Turn oven to 350°F and bake for 35 minutes. Once cooled, bread can be frozen if desired.

Nutritional Information (per slice):

- Calories: 130
- Fat: 2.6g
- Cholesterol: 0mg
- Sodium: 314mg
- Potassium: 128.8mg
- Carbohydrates: 24g
- Dietary Fiber: 3.4g
- Sugars: 2.3g
- Protein: 4.3g

Homemade Avocado Ranch

Prep Time: 10 minutes

Chill Time: 2 hours

Yield: 2 1/2 cups

Ingredients:

- 1 medium avocado
- 1/2 tsp. kosher salt
- 2 T. lime juice
- 3 T. buttermilk
- 1 c. low-sugar mayonnaise
- 1/2 c. plain Greek yogurt
- 2 T. chopped fresh cilantro leaves
- 2 T. dried parsley
- 2 tsp. onion powder
- 1 tsp. garlic powder
- 1 tsp. dried oregano
- 1/2 tsp. dried dill weed
- 1/2 tsp. black pepper

Directions:

Smash avocado with lime juice and salt. Slowly drizzle in buttermilk until the avocado mixture is thin enough to pour. More lime juice or buttermilk may be used if needed. Set aside. In a medium bowl or large measuring cup, whisk together mayonnaise and yogurt. Stir in cilantro and seasonings. Add avocado mixture and whisk until thoroughly combined. Chill for at least 2 hours before serving. Store in the refrigerator for up to a week.

Nutritional Information (per 1/4 cup):

- Calories: 83.5

- Fat: 3g

- Cholesterol: 1mg

- Sodium: 131.5mg

- Potassium: 143.2mg

- Carbohydrates: 13.4g

- Dietary Fiber: 1.6g

- Sugars: 10.5g

- Protein: 1.8g

Low-Sugar BBQ Sauce

Prep Time: 5 minutes

Cook Time: 30 minutes

Yield: 4 cups

Ingredients:

- 2 c. low-sugar ketchup
- 1/4 c. grated white onion
- 1/2 c. apple cider vinegar
- 1 c. beef broth
- 2 T. molasses
- 1 T. Worcestershire sauce
- 2 tsp. freshly ground black pepper
- 2 tsp. mustard
- 1/4 tsp. cayenne pepper
- 3-5 dashes hot sauce (optional)

Directions:

Bring all ingredients to a boil over medium heat. Reduce to low and simmer for 30 minutes, stirring occasionally.

Nutritional Information:

- Calories: 122.8
- Fat: 0g
- Cholesterol: 0mg
- Sodium: 164.7mg
- Potassium: 136.5mg
- Carbohydrates: 30g
- Dietary Fiber: 0.3g
- Sugars: 28.6g
- Protein: 0.5g

Carolina-Style Mustard BBQ Sauce

Prep Time: 5 minutes

Cook Time: 30 minutes

Yield: 2 cups

Ingredients:

- 1 c. yellow mustard
- 1/2 c. apple cider vinegar
- 3 T. dark brown sugar
- 2 T. Worcestershire sauce
- 1 T. chile powder
- 2 tsp. freshly ground black pepper
- 1 tsp. smoked paprika
- 3 dashes soy sauce

Directions:

Bring all ingredients to a boil over medium heat. Reduce to low and simmer for 30 minutes, stirring often. Be sure not to let the sauce scorch on the bottom of the pan. Serve with pork, ribs, or chicken.

Nutritional Information (per 1/4 cup):

- Calories: 48.3
- Fat: 1.1g
- Cholesterol: 0.4mg
- Sodium: 407.5mg
- Potassium: 128mg
- Carbohydrates: 9g
- Dietary Fiber: 1.7g
- Sugars: 5.5g
- Protein: 1.4g

Taco Seasoning

Prep Time: 5 minutes

Yield: 4 servings

Ingredients:

- 3 T. chile powder
- 1 T. ground cumin
- 1 tsp. paprika
- 1 tsp. smoked paprika
- 2 tsp. kosher salt
- 1 tsp. dried oregano
- 1 tsp. garlic powder
- 1 tsp. onion powder
- 1 tsp. dried oregano
- 1 tsp. black pepper
- 1 tsp. red pepper flakes
- 1 tsp. cornstarch

Directions:

Mix all ingredients and store in an airtight container for up to a month. To use, mix 2 tablespoons seasoning with each pound of taco meat. More or less seasoning can be used to taste.

Nutritional Information:

- Calories: 37
- Fat: 0.6g
- Cholesterol: 0mg
- Sodium: 1.1g
- Potassium: 137mg
- Carbohydrates: 7.9g
- Dietary Fiber: 1.9g
- Sugars: 0g
- Protein: 1.3g

Chocolate Nut Butter

Prep Time: 10 minutes

Yield: 2 cups

Ingredients:

- 1 c. hazelnuts (or other nuts), toasted
- 1 T. honey
- 1/2 lb. semisweet chocolate chips
- 2 T. butter
- 1/2 c. sweetened condensed milk

Directions:

Pulse nuts and honey in a food processor until a smooth paste forms. Melt the chocolate chips in a microwave-safe bowl by microwaving for about 2 minutes, stirring after every 20 seconds. Once the chocolate is melted, stir in the butter. Add sweetened condensed milk and stir until combined. Stream chocolate mixture into the food processor while blending until the hazelnut paste and chocolate are thoroughly combined.

Nutritional Information (per 1/4 cup):

- Calories: 285
- Fat: 22g
- Cholesterol: 9.1mg

- Sodium: 33.4mg
- Potassium: 240.5mg
- Carbohydrates: 23.8g
- Dietary Fiber: 3.3g
- Sugars: 19g
- Protein: 4.2g

Homemade Mayonnaise

Prep Time: 15 minutes

Yield: 2 cups

Ingredients:

- 2 egg yolks
- 1 tsp. ground mustard
- 1 tsp. kosher salt
- 1 T. white vinegar
- 2 T. lemon juice
- 2 c. canola oil

Directions:

Combine vinegar, lemon juice, and canola oil. Set aside. Whisk egg yolks, mustard, and salt in a medium bowl. Slowly drizzle in vinegar mixture while whisking. Be sure to add the mixture slowly to allow the mayonnaise to emulsify properly.

Nutritional Information (per 1/4 cup):

- Calories: 498.9
- Fat: 55.7g
- Cholesterol: 46mg
- Sodium: 292.6mg

- Potassium: 11.9mg
- Carbohydrates: 0.5g
- Dietary Fiber: 0g
- Sugars: 0.1g
- Protein: 0.8g

Chapter 5

Takeaways

1. Diabetes recipes can be delicious.
2. You can still eat many of your favorite foods with diabetes by making small adjustments to ingredients and portions.

One Last Thought

By some accounts, half of all Americans have been diagnosed with either diabetes or prediabetes. Learning to cook and plan meals that fit with a diabetes meal plan will help you and your loved ones live longer, healthier lives.

The two components of any healthy lifestyle are diet and exercise. Alongside physical activity, reducing the sugars in your diet can help your blood sugars remain stable. This book makes a great complement to your regular exercise program. Many of these recipes can be prepared in large batches on the weekend for easy meals throughout the workweek.

Why wait? You can make many of the recipes in this book without specialty ingredients or equipment.

Today is the best time to take control of your diet and your health!

By taking the time to learn to cook your favorite recipes in a diabetes-friendly way and evaluating which sugars your body absorbs most slowly, you can find increased energy and health. Using the recipes from this book, your entire family can enjoy tasty, delicious meals and snacks while you keep your diabetes under control.

Can You Help?

I'd love to hear your opinion about my book. In the world of book publishing, there are few things more valuable than honest reviews from a wide variety of readers.

Your review will help other readers find out if my book is for them. It will also help me reach more readers by increasing the visibility of my book.

Resources Cited

Davis PA & Yokoyama W (2011) Cinnamon intake lowers fasting blood glucose: meta analysis. J Med Food 14:884-889.

"Diabetes Latest." National Center for Chronic Disease Prevention and Health Promotion, 2014: https://www.cdc.gov/features/diabetesfactsheet/

Ejtahed HS, Mohtadi-Nia J, Homayouni-Rad A, Niafar M, Asghari-Jafarabadi M, & Mofid V (2012) Probiotic yogurt improves antioxidant status in type 2 diabetes patients. Nutrition 28:539-543.

Kassaian N, Azadbakht L, Forghani B, & Amini M (2009) Effect of fenugreek seeds on blood glucose and lipid profiles in type 2 diabetes patients. Int J Vitam Nutr Res 79: 34-39.

Sharma RD, Raghuram TC, & Rao NS (1990) Effect of fenugreek seeds on blood glucose and serum lipids in type 1 diabetes. Eur J Clin Nutr 44:301-306.

Made in the USA
San Bernardino, CA
21 May 2018